18.99

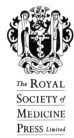

The ROYAL
SOCIETY *of*
MEDICINE
PRESS *Limited*

Female Urinary Incontinence in Practice

Matthew Parsons
Clinical Research Fellow in
Urogynaecology, King's College
Hospital, London

Linda Cardozo
Professor of Urogynaecology and
Consultant Gynaecologist, King's
College Hospital, London

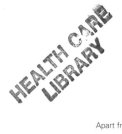

© 2004 Royal Society of Medicine Press Ltd
Published by the Royal Society of Medicine Press Ltd
1 Wimpole Street, London W1G 0AE, UK
Tel: +44 (0) 20 7290 2921
Fax: +44 (0) 20 7290 2929
E-mail: publishing@rsm.ac.uk
Website: www.rsmpress.co.uk

The authors are responsible for the scientific content and for the views expressed, which are not necessarily those of the Royal Society of Medicine or of the Royal Society of Medicine Press Ltd.

Although every effort has been made to ensure that, where provided, information concerning drug dosages or product usage has been presented accurately in this publication, the ultimate responsibility rests with the prescribing physician and neither the publisher nor the sponsor can be held responsible for errors or any consequences arising from the use of information contained herein.

British Library Cataloguing in Publication Data

A catalogue record for this book is available from the British Library

ISBN 1 85315 581 0
ISSN 1473 6845

Distribution in Europe and Rest of World:
Marston Book Services Ltd
PO Box 269
Abingdon
Oxon OX14 4YN, UK
Tel: +44 (0) 1235 465500
Fax: +44 (0) 1235 465555

Distribution in the USA and Canada:
Royal Society of Medicine Press Ltd
c/o Jamco Distribution Inc.
1401 Lakeway Drive
Lewisville TX 75057, USA
Tel: +1 800 538 1287
Fax: +1 972 353 1303
E-mail: jamco@majors.com

Distribution in Australia and New Zealand:
Elsevier Australia
30–52 Smidmore Street
Marrickville NSW 2204
Australia
Tel: + 61 2 9517 8999
Fax: + 61 2 9517 2249
E-mail: service@elsevier.com.au

Typeset by Phoenix Photosetting, Chatham, Kent
Printed in Great Britain by Latimer Trend & Company Ltd, Plymouth

About the authors

Matthew Parsons is Clinical Research Fellow in the Department of Urogynaecology at King's College Hospital, London. He trained at the University of Bristol, graduating MB ChB in 1993. Mr Parsons passed the MRCOG in 2000 and was awarded a Certificate of Completion of Specialist Training (CCST) in Obstetrics and Gynaecology in June 2003.

He developed his interest in urogynaecology while working for Professor Cardozo as a Senior House Officer and elected to undertake special-interest training after CCST. Mr Parsons has interests in all aspects of urogynaecology, including management of intractable interstitial cystitis, normal voiding function and use of a computerized bladder diary in the assessment of lower urinary tract dysfunction. He works as part of a multidisciplinary team in a busy tertiary referral urogynaecology department under the guidance of Professor Cardozo.

Linda Cardozo is Professor of Urogynaecology and Consultant Gynaecologist at King's College Hospital, London. She trained at Liverpool University Medical School and qualified MB ChB in 1974. Thereafter she developed a special interest in urinary incontinence at St George's Hospital under the aegis of Professor Stuart Stanton, obtaining an MD in 1979 and the MRCOG in 1980.

Following her appointment as a Consultant Obstetrician and Gynaecologist in 1985, she continued to develop her interest in all aspects of urogynaecology, including the influence of hormones on the lower urinary tract, conservative and surgical treatment of stress incontinence, the pathophysiology and pharmacological treatment of detrusor overactivity, and the management of urogenital prolapse.

Professor Cardozo is now the head of a busy and productive tertiary referral urogynaecology department at King's College Hospital. She has a large clinical workload, dealing with complex urogynaecological problems in a supra-regional tertiary referral unit, teaching medical students, training junior doctors and undertaking clinical research. Her publications include more than 200 original papers in peer review journals and 9 books.

Professor Cardozo is Chairman of the British Society of Urogynaecology, Chairman of the Continence Foundation UK and President of the Association of Chartered Physiotherapists in Women's Health. She is also Past President of the International Urogynaecological Association, Past President of the Section of Obstetrics and Gynaecology of the Royal Society of Medicine and Past Chairman of the British Menopause Society. In addition, Professor Cardozo is a fellows representative on the Council of the Royal College of Obstetricians and Gynaecologists and Chairman of the Education Committee of the International Continence Society as well as Vice Chairman of the World Health Organization International Consultation on Incontinence.

Preface

Urinary incontinence (UI) is a common distressing condition that affects millions of men and women worldwide. It is defined by the International Continence Society (ICS) as 'any involuntary leakage of urine'. In population estimates, the range for urinary leakage varies, but only a minority perceive it as a problem – using the original ICS definition of 'involuntary urinary leakage that is a social or hygienic problem'. Urinary incontinence may be the endpoint of multiple pathological processes.

Urogynaecology encompasses problems of the female lower urinary tract and genital tract. Because they are in close proximity to each other, they often develop co-existent disorders. Although rarely life-threatening, urinary problems (such as incontinence and pelvic organ prolapse) cause distress to the individual or her carers, significantly impair quality of life and impose a considerable financial burden on the healthcare budget of the nation.

Sufferers may have to alter many of their routines and habits. This can be detrimental to their social lives, relationships, job and psychological well-being. Daily routines and chores are planned around the known location of toilets, and avoidance behaviour ensues because of anxiety about public embarrassment and fears of humiliation. Problems are often hidden even from spouses, and social isolation and relationship problems may develop.

By improving diagnosis of these common conditions, management can be appropriately targeted. This will reduce morbidity and allow otherwise healthy women to lead normal active lives.

Incontinence has probably been a problem since prehistoric times but there was little interest in investigating the aetiology and potential treatment of UI until the 18th Century. Many different surgical techniques were developed, although with no understanding of or means to investigate the underlying causes, early continence surgery met with little success.

Cystometry, the measurement of the pressure–volume relationship of the bladder, was pioneered in 1882 by Mosso and Pellicani using a smoke drum and water manometer.[1] Along with air cystoscopy (developed by Kelly in 1893), they formed the beginnings of a classification system for incontinence.[1] As technology improved further the appreciation of the potential mechanisms of incontinence became better. In 1964 Enhorning, Miller and Hinman combined cystometry with radiographic screening of the bladder, and in 1971 Bates, Turner-Warwick and Whiteside introduced synchronous cine pressure–flow cystography with pressure and flow-studies. This was the beginning of the field of videourodynamics. Hodgkinson described 'dyssynergic detrusor dysfunction' in 1963, recognizing the importance of diagnosing it prior to incontinence surgery. Bates and Turner-Warwick developed the understanding of abnormal detrusor activity and coined the term 'detrusor instability', so that the role of abnormal detrusor activity as a cause of incontinence was fully appreciated and treatment became more coordinated.[2]

However, the correlation between symptoms and urodynamic diagnosis is poor, and it remains essential to make an accurate diagnosis because the treatments for various underlying causative conditions are so different. Treatment ranges from simple lifestyle advice and behavioural modification, to physical and pharmacological therapies, to complex and potentially difficult surgical intervention. It is not always possible to cure, but much can be done to improve or manage the problem.

This book is aimed at everyone with an interest in treating women with urinary incontinence, especially primary-care doctors and nurses. Initial investigation and treatment is perfectly reasonable in the primary-care setting. It may prove to be very successful prior to referral to a gynaecologist, urogynaecologist or urologist (if necessary).

M Parsons
L Cardozo

References

1. Bidmead J, Cardozo L. Short cuts. In Sturdee D, Oláh K, Purdie D, Keane D (eds). *Yearbook of Obstetrics and Gynaecology – Volume 10*. London: RCOG Press, 2002.

2. Drutz HP, Schulz JA. History of urogynaecology. In Staskin D, Cardozo LD (eds). *Textbook of Female Urology and Urogynaecology*. Oxford: Isis Medical Media, 2001, pp 215–26.

Acknowledgements

We are grateful for the help of Kate Anders, Senior Nurse Specialist; Dudley Robinson, Clinical Fellow; and James Balmforth, Subspecialty Trainee, Department of Urogynaecology, King's College Hospital, for their help in writing chapters and for their advice and suggestions on the writing of this book.

Contents

1. Background – the scope of the problem

Prevalence
Risk factors – race
Risk factors – cognitive and
  psychiatric disorders
Financial burden

Prevalence

In population estimates the prevalence of urinary incontinence (UI) varies from 10% to 40%.[1] However, only 7–12% perceive it as a problem.[2] Studies of incidence and prevalence of UI are hampered by the heterogeneous definitions of urinary incontinence applied by different researchers in different countries. The International Continence Society defines UI as 'any involuntary leakage of urine'.[3] However, epidemiological studies often use a 'frequency' definition, eg more than two episodes in a month.[4] Prevalence, the likelihood of detecting a given condition within a defined population at a specific point in time, is important for planning and allocating healthcare resources. This should not be confused with incidence, which is the likelihood of developing a

condition during a given time period – usually 1-, 2- or 5-year intervals.

> The ICS defines incontinence as 'any involuntary leakage of urine'

The EPINCONT study

In the Norwegian EPINCONT community-based survey, 25% of all respondents had some urinary leakage, the prevalence being age-dependent (Figure 1.1).[1]

Of the women studied:

- 50% complained of stress incontinence
- 11% had urge
- 36% had mixed incontinence.[1]

Smaller studies based in local communities support these high rates. At one general practice in Bristol, UK, the prevalence of UI was 53%.[5] It is likely that most studies underestimate the prevalence of UI in populations due to reporting bias, and it is essential that this is addressed in epidemiological surveys.[6]

The prevalence of UI peaks at 45–55 years of age, dips slightly thereafter, and increases again after age 70.[7] This may be due to diminishing stress incontinence (Figure 1.2).[1] It may be accompanied by an increasing incidence of detrusor overactivity or overactive bladder,

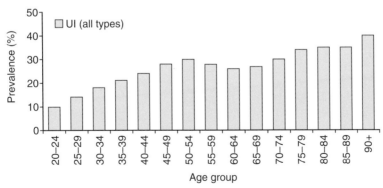

Figure 1
Prevalence of all urinary incontinence (UI) in the EPINCONT study (*n* = 27 936)

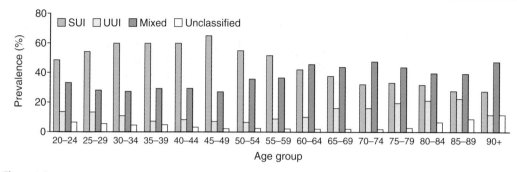

Figure 1.2
The prevalence of symptoms according to age in the EPINCONT study (*n* = 6792). SUI, stress urinary incontinence; UUI, urge urinary incontinence

which have been shown to increase linearly with age (Figure 1.3).[8]

> Detrusor overactivity and overactive bladder increase linearly with age

Risk factors – race

During an analysis of 183 African–Americans and 132 Caucasians referred consecutively for bothersome lower urinary tract symptoms, pelvic organ prolapse or both, stepwise logistic regression was used to compare risk factors for incontinence. Caucasian race was the most significant predictor of urodynamic stress incontinence [relative risk (RR) 2.21, confidence interval (CI) 1.31–3.73], and African–American race was the only significant predictor of detrusor overactivity (RR 2.6, CI 1.45–4.80).[9] There was no significant difference in type or severity of prolapse in this study.

Risk factors – cognitive and psychiatric disorders

In addition to the general population, urinary symptoms are frequently found in institutionalized women and those with psychiatric disorders. In 1995 a working party of The Royal College of Physicians reported that incontince was suffered by:

- 15% of women living at home
- 25% of women in residential care
- 40% of women in nursing homes
- 60% of women in long-term hospital care.[10]

The prevalence of UI is high in women with psychiatric disorders and those who are institutionalized, possibly because these women are more impaired and more dependent

> Prevalence has always been higher in institutionalized women, probably because they tend to be more dependent and more impaired.

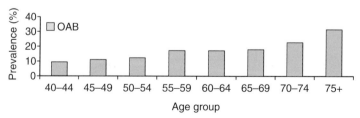

Figure 1.3
The prevalence of overactive bladder (OAB) symptoms by age in a European population survey (*n* = 16 776)

Conversely, existing UI increases the risk of admission to hospital (RR 1.3, CI 1.2–1.5) and to long-term care (RR 2.0, CI 1.7–2.4) when age and co-morbid conditions are controlled.[11] In a sample of 100 elderly patients suffering from cognitive impairment, 35% were found to have UI.[12]

Psychiatric disorders causing incontinence have not been well studied. However, major depression and panic disorder are highly prevalent in women with UI – 16% and 7%, respectively.[13] Patients with urge and mixed UI are significantly more likely to have coexistent psychiatric illness. Co-morbid major depression significantly impacts on a patient's UI symptom reporting, incontinence-specific quality-of-life and functional status. Depression also occurs in other conditions associated with urge incontinence, such as ageing and dementia. The nature of this relationship may not be causal, but rather a common pathology.

Depression often occurs alongside urinary incontinence

Financial burden

The annual economic cost of managing UI in the UK has been estimated at £354 million.[14] The Continence Foundation (see Appendix C) has conservatively estimated treatment costs in England for 1998.[15] The local area cost can be calculated by multiplying the local population in thousands by the appropriate figure given in Table 1.1.

Table 1.1
The economic cost of incontinence estimated for England in 1998

	Actual cost (£ million)	Cost/1000 population (£)
Drugs	22 732	467
Appliances	58 612	1189
Containment products	69 000	1400
Staff costs and direct overheads	189 926	3814
Surgery	13 325	270
Minimum total	353 595	7178

The costs of drugs and appliances have been updated and the Continence Foundation has published new figures for 1999 (Table 1.2).[16]

Table 1.2
Drugs and appliances costs for 1999

DRUGS 1999	Prescription items dispensed (thousands)	NIC (£)	Cost/item dispensed (£)	Change from 1998 in items dispensed	Change from 1998 in NIC
TOTAL	1502.7	26 888 700	17.89	+16.7%	+37.2%
Add 16% for dispensing cost *		31 190 800			+37.2%
APPLIANCES 1999	Prescription items dispensed (thousands)	NIC (£)	Cost/item dispensed (£)	Change from 1998 in items dispensed	Change from 1998 in NIC
TOTAL	1629.9	54 453 100	33.41	+4.8%	+7.8%
Add 16% for dispensing cost *		63 165 600			+7.8%

* Advised by NHSE Pharmacy & Prescribing Branch Source: *Prescription Cost Analysis – England – 1999* (Department of Health, 2000)
NIC, net ingredient cost

This represents a significant increase in the expenditure on prescribed drugs and appliances, which presumably will increase each year.

References

1. Hannestad YS, Rortveit G, Sandvik H, Hunskaar S. A community-based epidemiological survey of female urinary incontinence: the Norwegian EPINCONT study. Epidemiology of incontinence in the County of Nord-Trondelag. *J Clin Epidemiol* 2000; **53:** 1150–7.

2. McGrowther CW, Shaw C, Perry SI *et al.* Epidemiology (Europe). In Cardozo L, Staskin D (eds). *Textbook of Female Urology and Urogynaecology.* Oxford: Isis Medical Media, 2001; pp 21–35.

3. Abrams P, Cardozo L, Fall M *et al.* The standardisation of Terminology of Lower Urinary Tract Function: Report from the Standardisation Sub-Committee of the International Continence Society. *Neurourol Urodyn* 2002; **21:** 167–78.

4. Hunskaar S, Burgio K, Diokno A *et al.* Epidemiology and natural history of urinary incontinence in women. *Urology* 2003; **62 (Suppl 4A):** 16–23.

5. Harrison GL, Memel DS. Urinary incontinence in women; its prevalence and its management in a health promotion clinic. *Br J Gen Pract* 1994; **44:** 147–8.

6. Fultz NH, Herzog AR. Prevalence of urinary incontinence in middle-aged and older women: a survey-based methodological experiment. *J Aging Health* 2000; **12:** 459–69.

7. Thomas TM, Plymat KR, Blannin J, Meade TW. Prevalence of urinary incontinence. *Br Med J* 1980; **281:** 1243–5.

8. Milsom I, Abrams P, Cardozo L *et al.* How widespread are the symptoms of overactive bladder and how are they managed? A population-based prevalence study. *BJU Int* 2001; **87:** 760–6.

9. Graham CA, Mallett VT. Race as a predictor of urinary incontinence and pelvic organ prolapse. *Am J Obstet Gynecol* 2001; **185:** 116–20.

10. Anonymous. Incontinence. Causes, management and provision of services. A Working Party of the Royal College of Physicians. *J R Coll of Phys Lond* 1995; **29:** 272–4.

11. Thom DH, Haan MN, van den Eeden S. Medically recognised urinary incontinence and risk of hospitalisation, nursing home admission, and mortality. *Age Ageing* 1997; **26:** 367–74.

12. Berrios GE. Urinary Incontinence and the Psychopathology of the Elderly with Cognitive Failure. *Gerontology* 1986; **32:** 119–24.

13. Melville JL, Walker E, Katon W *et al.* Prevalence of co-morbid psychiatric illness and its impact on symptom perception, quality of life, and functional status in women with urinary incontinence. *Am J Obstet Gynaecol* 2002; **187:** 80–7.

14. Department of Health. *Modernising Health and Social Services: National Priorities Guidance. 1999/00–2001/02.* London: Department of Health, 1998.

15. The Continence Foundation. The Cost of Incontinence to the NHS. (http://www.continence-foundation.org.uk/ in-depth/integrated-continence-service.php#13)

16. Department of Helath. *Prescription Cost Analysis – England, 1999. Continence Foundation Newsletter* 2001; **issue 6**.

2. Structural development

Introduction
Embryology
Physiology
Anatomy

Introduction

The lower urinary tract in human adult females is comprised of the bladder and urethra, which act together with the pelvic floor structures as a single functional unit (Figure 2.1).

> The female lower urinary tract is made up of the bladder, urethra and pelvic floor structures

Embryology

The inner cell mass of the blastocyst develops into a bilaminar germ disc after implanting in the uterine cavity. The ectodermal cells are continuous with amnioblasts and surround the amniotic cavity. Endodermal cells are continuous with the exocoelomic membrane and surround the yolk sac. Mesoderm subsequently separates them to form the trilaminar germ disc. This occurs by the third week of development. During the embryonic period, from the fourth to eighth week of intrauterine life, lateral and cephalocaudal folding occurs, as does organogenesis in each of the three germ cell layers.

Formation of the tube-like gut is a passive process consisting of inversion and incorporation of the yolk sac into the body cavity. The hindgut is formed in the tail region, where a small diverticulum (called the allantois) is located. The part of the allantois connected to the hindgut is called the cloaca. The hindgut ends, temporarily, at the cloacal membrane (see Figure 2.2).

Division of the cloaca occurs. This is caused by the downward growth of a ridge of mesenchymal tissue, called the urorectal septum (Figure 2.3). Therefore an anterior part (the primitive bladder and urogenital membrane) and a posterior part (the anorectal canal and anal membrane) are formed.

> The cloaca divides to form the anterior part (primitive bladder and urogenital membrane) and the posterior part (anorectal canal and anal membrane)

Development of the kidneys

Development of the kidneys occurs in the mesenchymal tissue, during three overlapping phases:

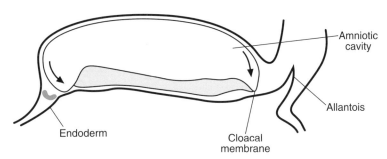

Figure 2.1
The flat bilaminar germ disc

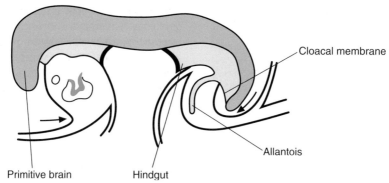

Figure 2.2
Folding of the germ disc to form the body cavity

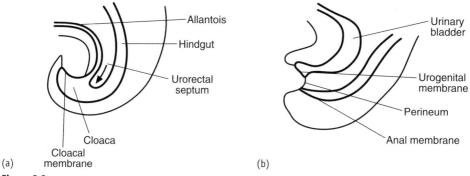

Figure 2.3
(a) Downgrowth of the urorectal septum. (b) Division of the cloaca into anterior and posterior parts

- The first stage, the pronephros, consists of 10 cell clusters and is non-functional.
- The mesonephros develops on each side and forms a large ovoid structure projecting into the abdominal (coelomic) cavity.
- The primitive gonads are found on the medial aspect of this ovoid structure, known as the urogenital ridge. Its tubules open into a collecting system called the mesonephric duct (Figure 2.4). Although it functions as a primitive kidney, it disappears completely in the female.

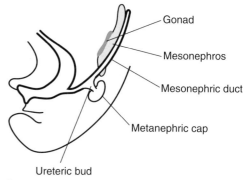

Figure 2.4
Mesonephros and mesonephric duct, showing ureteric bud

The three phases of kidney development in the mesenchymal tissue are:

- the pronephros
- the mesonephros
- the metanephros

In males testosterone stimulates the mesonephric duct to develop into the epididymis and vas deferens.

The permanent kidney is derived from the metanephros, which develops in the fifth week. The excretory units form from the metanephric (mesodermal) cap. The collecting system is formed by the ureteric bud, an out-branching of the mesonephric duct, near its entrance into the cloaca.

The caudal part of the mesonephric duct is absorbed into the primitive bladder (Figure 2.5), and so the ureteric duct is drawn in. With growth of the bladder, the ureteric ducts move laterally and the mesonephric ducts come to lie in close proximity to each other, caudal to the ureteric bud where the primitive bladder will become the urethra.

The growth of the bladder causes the mesonephric ducts to move closer together, caudal to the ureteric bud where the primitive bladder will develop in to the urethra

The trigone (a triangular area of the bladder bound by the ureteric orifices and the internal urethral meatus) will develop from the tissues derived from the mesonephric duct (Figure 2.6), and is therefore of mesodermal origin. The upper part of the bladder is of endodermal origin, having been derived from the yolk sac.

Müllerian ducts

Müllerian ducts develop in to the main genital tract in females, but regress in males

Both male and female embryos initially have a further pair of genital ducts known as the Müllerian ducts. These arise from an invagination of the epithelium on the antero-lateral surface of the urogenital ridge. They develop into the main genital duct in the female, forming:

- uterus
- fallopian tubes
- cervix
- upper vagina.

(Under the influence of Müllerian inhibiting substance, produced by the Sertoli cells in the testes, the Müllerian ducts regress in the male.)

The most caudal part of the cloaca is of endodermal origin. It is known as the urogenital sinus and forms the distal vagina and urethra.

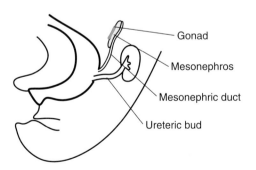

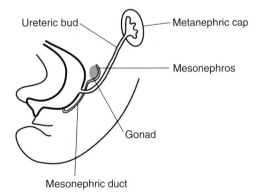

Figure 2.5
Reabsorption of the mesonephric duct draws in the ureteric bud

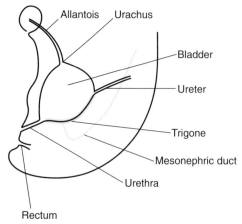

Figure 2.6
Embryology of the lower urinary tract by eight weeks

Thus, the fallopian tubes, uterus, cervix, and trigone appear to have a common embryological mesodermal origin. The upper bladder and lower parts of the vagina and urethra have a common endodermal origin. Full development of the lower urinary tract occurs by the 12th week of intrauterine life.

> By the 12th week of intrauterine life, the lower urinary tract has fully developed

Physiology

The bladder wall is made up of both elastic and contractile elements, reflecting its dual function. These elements include:

- smooth muscle
- collagen
- elastin.

Additionally, there are vascular and nervous components and transitional cell epithelium.

The bladder functions as a reservoir where urine is stored during the filling phase. This requires it to be a compliant organ, so that intravesical pressure shows minimal change as the stored volume increases. Intravesical pressure must remain low so that filling may

continue from the upper tracts, and also to prevent urethral closure pressure being overcome, which would result in urine leakage per urethram.

Filling of bladder

The bladder fills physiologically at 0.5–5 ml/minute. The sensation of bladder filling is conveyed via afferent nerves travelling with the thoraco-lumbar (T10–L2) and sacral (S2–4) efferent nerves.

> The bladder fills at a rate of 0.5–5 ml per minute

As the bladder fills with urine, the detrusor muscle is relaxed and the urethral sphincter is contracted in order to maintain continence. The detrusor muscle is innervated by the cholinergic parasympathetic nerves (which cause contraction of the muscle) and β-sympathetic nerves (which result in bladder relaxation).[1] Cholinergic and non-cholinergic transmitters are involved. Evidence also exists that neuropeptide-releasing ganglion cells are present in the innervation of the bladder.[2] The intrinsic urethral sphincter (rhabdosphincter) and extrinsic urethral sphincter (levator ani muscle complex) are supplied by somatic nerves derived from S2–4. Fibres travelling to the rhabdosphincter do so via the pelvic splanchnic nerves, and those innervating the levator ani do so via the perineal branch of the pudendal nerve.

Control of voiding

Central control of micturition is via the sacral spinal reflex. Inhibition of micturition comes from the cerebral cortex, cerebellum, and subcortex including the hypothalamus, thalamus, basal ganglia, limbic system and pontine reticular formation.

When voiding is initiated, inhibition of sympathetic activity results in urethral relaxation. The rhabdosphincter and levator ani are under voluntary control and are consciously relaxed. Inhibition of the voiding reflex by the cortical centres is then repressed and detrusor contraction occurs due to unopposed parasympathetic activity.[3]

Continence requires normal urinary tract anatomy accompanied by intact neurological pathways. Infants do not have voluntary control of micturition – cortical inhibition of reflex bladder activity is learned with toilet training. For this to be learned successfully, there must be sufficient neurological development.

> Continence is a learned activity, requiring intact neurological pathways and a normal urinary tract anatomy

Continence during filling requires:

- adequate bladder compliance
- an effective urethral sphincter
- a developed, intact nervous system.

Low-level afferent activity in the pelvic and pudendal nerves leads to reflex efferent activity in the sympathetic and somatic pathways to the bladder and urethra. Parasympathetic activity is suppressed. During exertion, eg running, the role of the sphincter mechanism becomes even more important, as does the correct positioning of the proximal urethra (which should be intra-abdominal) and the resistance offered by urethral mucosal coaptation.

For micturition to occur there must be repression of the cortical inhibition of the voiding reflex and relaxation of the urethral sphincter. This again requires intact neurological tracts and is achieved by the inhibition of sympathetic and somatic pathways by vesical afferent fibres, allowing the parasympathetic nerves to predominate.

Anatomy

The urinary bladder is an extraperitoneal organ situated behind the pubic bones. It is a strong, muscular receptacle for the storage of urine. Its shape when empty differs markedly from its shape when full.

Empty bladder

The empty bladder is pyramidal in shape. Its apex is behind the upper margin of the symphysis pubis and is attached to the umbilicus by the urachus (a remnant of the obliterated allantois), which passes upwards in the extraperitoneal fat to form the median umbilical ligament. The base of the pyramid is triangular and is formed by the trigone. The two superior corners are formed by the entrance of the ureters, which enter obliquely through the bladder wall. The inferior corner is formed by the urethral entrance/bladder neck. The superior surface of the bladder is entirely covered with peritoneum and lies in close proximity to the uterovesical pouch and the body of the uterus. The inferolateral surfaces are related to, ie adjacent to, the retropubic fat pad and the pubic bones. Posteriorly, they are also close to the obturator internus muscle and the levator ani muscle. The bladder neck rests on the upper surface of the urogenital diaphragm, where it is held in position by the pubovesical ligaments; see Figure 2.7.

Full bladder

As the bladder fills, the superior surface of the bladder is pushed out to form an ovoid structure that projects above the symphysis pubis. The posterior surface and bladder neck remain in essentially the same position.

The mucous membrane that covers the majority of the bladder is thrown into folds when the bladder is empty. These folds then disappear when the bladder is full. The membrane overlying the base of the bladder, the trigone, is always smooth as the connective tissue is strongly adherent to the underlying muscle. The muscular layer of the bladder is known as the detrusor and is arranged as three layers of interlacing muscle fibres. Contraction of this muscular mesh results in a reduction in the bladder size in all dimensions. The smooth muscle of the trigone has only two layers,

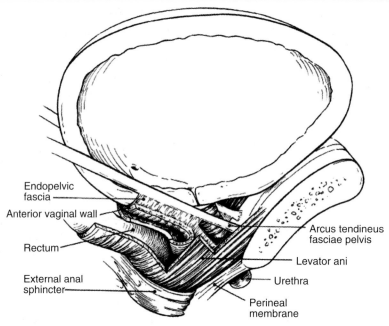

Figure 2.7
General anatomy of the lower urinary tract. Adapted with permission from John DeLancey

which are less well developed than other areas of the bladder.

References

1. Khanna OMP. Disorders of micturition: neurophysiological basis and results of drug therapy. *Urology* 1986; **136**: 1022.

2. Mundy AR. Neuropeptides in lower urinary tract function. *World J Urol* 1984; **2**: 211–15.

3. Tanagho EA, Miller ER. Initiation of voiding. *Br J Urol* 1970; **42**: 175–83.

3. Assessment

History
Physical examination
Quality-of-life assessment
Investigations
Specialist investigations
Ambulatory urodynamics
Imaging of the urinary tract
Conclusion

History

The worldwide ageing of the population is likely to increase the burden of incontinence on health services. It will be increasingly necessary for all doctors to treat incontinence to some extent. Symptoms can be due to a wide variety of underlying aetiological mechanisms and it is therefore important to approach assessment in a logical and objective manner.

> The ageing of the population is likely to increase the incontinence-related costs and burden on the health services

An accurate and detailed history and examination provide a framework for diagnosis. However, it is important to recognize that different underlying conditions can cause similar urinary symptoms and that medical history alone is a poor predictor of pathophysiology. Diagnosis based on history has been shown to have a sensitivity of 77.9% and a specificity of only 38.7% in women complaining of urgency and urge incontinence.[1] The principal mechanisms of stress incontinence, urge incontinence and associated irritative bladder symptoms and overflow incontinence should be borne in mind when taking a history.

Definitions

Stress urinary incontinence (SUI) is the complaint of involuntary leakage of urine on effort or exertion, or on sneezing or coughing. It is the commonest presenting symptom for which women seek advice.

> Stress urinary incontinence is the most common symptom that causes women to seek advice from their doctor. USI is the involuntary leakage of urine on effort or exertion

Urge urinary incontinence is the complaint of involuntary leakage accompanied by, or immediately preceded by, a strong desire to void.

Symptom categories

The International Continence Society has published several new symptom categories. Mixed incontinence is the complaint of involuntary leakage associated with urgency and with exertion, effort, sneezing or coughing. *Nocturnal enuresis* is the complaint of loss of urine during sleep. (Enuresis is any involuntary loss of urine.) Continuous urinary incontinence is the complaint of continuous leakage, classically associated with a fistula or urethral diverticulum. *Situational incontinence* may be reported, eg giggle incontinence.[2]

Urological symptoms

Urological symptoms may not be accurate when used alone in the diagnosis of urinary incontinence (UI). They do, however, give important clues to the diagnosis and can be used to help monitor the effects of subsequent treatment. The onset of urinary symptoms and their duration and severity should be recorded. Symptoms of detrusor overactivity (DO) should be assessed:

- frequency
- urgency
- urge incontinence
- nocturia.

Symptoms of detrusor overactivity include urgency, frequency, nocturia and urge incontinence

One should also enquire about the presence of stress incontinence, urinary tract infections and voiding difficulty. Nocturnal enuresis as a child is often associated with DO as an adult. A history of previous urological investigations, their result and any ensuing treatment, especially of incontinence surgery, is very important to note.

It is very important to take a full medical history when diagnosing a lower urinary tract disorder

Coexisting conditions

If women complain of incontinence it is important to check for coexistent medical conditions and optimize their treatment. For example, the onset of diabetes significantly increases urine output and many pharmaceutical agents can alter bladder function. In order to gain an accurate impression of the psychosocial morbidity associated with the patient's condition, it is important to elucidate the restrictions it brings to everyday life and the coping strategies adopted to deal with these restrictions.

Many women complain of persistent urinary problems after pregnancy and childbirth. On closer questioning irritative bladder symptoms may have been present for several years prior to the pregnancy in those women found to have DO. However, both stress and urge incontinence may arise de novo at any time, especially after delivery.[3, 4]

Physical examination

Abdominal and pelvic examination form an essential part of the assessment of any woman who presents with urinary incontinence. If there are any symptoms that point to a possible neurological cause, it is important to perform a screening neurological examination.

The patient's mobility and mental state affect her ability to react to her symptoms, and it may be appropriate to formally test these as part of the examination as they will influence management. Similarly, an assessment of motivation and manual dexterity is important in determining the treatment most likely to prove effective.

An abdominal and pelvic examination should form part of the assessment, as should a screening neurological examination if it is thought that there might be a neurological cause

Pelvic organ prolapse

Because of the close proximity of the lower urinary and genital tracts in the female, the presence of pelvic organ prolapse can have an important bearing on urinary symptoms and their management. The grade of prolapse can be classified subjectively as mild, moderate or severe or graded according to the International Continence Society (ICS) pelvic organ prolapse quantification score (POP-Q).[5]

A cystocele may cause urgency and frequency as it drags on the trigone and causes messages of bladder fullness to be sent to the brain

A cystocele, which drags on the trigone of the bladder, may give rise to urgency and frequency as the trigone stretches and afferent fibres convey a sense of bladder fullness to the brain. Excursion of the bladder neck during coughing may lead to stress incontinence. This is often (but not exclusively) associated with anterior vaginal wall prolapse when a deficiency or abnormality in tissue collagen may be a common aetiological factor. In addition, pelvic masses, such as ovarian cysts or uterine enlargement, can cause urinary symptoms, and these conditions need to be excluded by bimanual examination. If this cannot be done with confidence, for example in the obese patient, then a transvaginal ultrasound scan should be considered.

Quality-of-life assessment

The impairment of quality of life (QoL) caused by urinary incontinence is difficult to predict using symptoms and urodynamic studies alone. In addition, individuals vary greatly in their perception of the significance of their lower urinary tract symptoms and how severely these restrict their normal psychosocial function. QoL questionnaires are therefore a useful adjunct in assessing the impact of urinary incontinence and bladder dysfunction.

> QoL questionnaires are useful in assessing the impact that incontinence and bladder dysfunction have on a woman's life

In 1978 the World Health Organization defined health as 'not merely the absence of disease, but complete physical, mental and social wellbeing'.[6] It has been suggested that the assessment of QoL should include:

- those attributes valued by patients, including their resultant comfort or sense of well-being
- the extent to which they are able to maintain reasonable physical, emotional and intellectual function
- the degree to which they retain their ability to participate in valued activities within the family and the community'.[7]

This helps to emphasize the multidimensional nature of QoL and the importance of considering the patient's own perception of her situation regarding non-health-related aspects of her life.[8]

There are many validated questionnaires available to assess QoL impairment [eg King's Health Questionnaire, Bristol Female Lower Urinary Tract Symptom Questionnaire (BFLUTS), Incontinence Impact Questionnaire (IIQ), Urogenital Distress Inventory (UDI)] due to urinary disorders. Most of these have a similar structure, consisting of a series of sections (domains) designed to gather information regarding particular aspects of health. They are particularly helpful for monitoring response to treatment. The King's

Health Questionnaire is a validated and reliable, disease-specific quality-of-life questionnaire that is freely available to all healthcare professionals for use in everyday practice (see Appendix A).

Investigations

Urinary symptom analysis alone is not sufficient to gain an accurate impression of the underlying pathology, as this may lead to inappropriate treatment being given. Even simple office investigations (Table 3.1) may be invaluable in identifying associated causal factors not immediately apparent:

- Culture of the urine may identify urinary tract infection (UTI).
- Urinalysis may aid in detection of UTI and diabetes mellitus.
- Post-void residual check (either by ultrasound scan or catheterization) excludes overflow incontinence.
- A frequency–volume chart may identify the compulsive fluid drinker, or those drinking excessive alcohol and caffeine.

> Investigations such as urine culture, urinalysis, post-voidal residual check and frequency–volume charts may help identify causal factors

See inside front cover flowchart.

Table 3.1
Investigations of lower urinary tract symptoms

Basic investigations	Midstream urine specimen
	Frequency–volume chart
	Post-void residual
	Pad test
Specialist investigations	Uroflowmetry
	Subtracted cystometry
	Videourodynamics
	Ambulatory urodynamics
	Urethral pressure profilometry
	Leak-point pressures
	Ultrasonography
	Radiological imaging
	Cystoscopy

Urine culture

The symptoms of DO overlap with those of UTI. In either case the patient may complain of:

- frequency and/or urgency of micturition
- only passing small volumes of urine
- a constant desire to pass urine.

The presence of UTI will worsen irritative bladder symptoms and invalidate the results of urodynamic investigations. A pure growth of more than 100 000 organisms/ml of urine is taken to signify infection that should be treated with appropriate antibiotics.[9] Recurrent UTI requires investigation to ensure that the bladder is completely emptied after each void. Investigations will also exclude the presence of any focus for infection, such as ureteric or intravesical calculi, or neoplasm.

Frequency–volume chart

The frequency–volume (FV) chart (Figure 3.1) is an important tool in the investigation of patients with lower urinary tract symptoms and voiding dysfunction.[10] The chart is variously known as a FV chart, bladder diary or voiding diary, and is completed daily by the patient over a number of days prior to the visit to the doctor. This facilitates history taking regarding the degree of frequency, nocturia and volumes voided at each episode. Compulsive or excessive fluid consumption, normal consumption at inappropriate times (eg bedtime), or an excessive intake of alcohol or caffeine is easily identified and behavioural modification can be commenced (Table 3.2).

Functional bladder capacity should be consistently around 300–500 ml. Frequent voids of variable amounts throughout the day imply bladder overactivity or behavioural adaptation to symptoms.

> Functional bladder capacity should stay at a steady level of 300–500 ml

The FV chart has been shown to be a valuable, reliable tool for the assessment of voiding

Table 3.2

Information that can be derived from a frequency–volume chart

- Functional bladder capacity
- A volumetric summary of diurnal urinary frequency
- A volumetric summary of nocturnal urinary frequency
- Quantification of total fluid intake
- Distribution and type of fluid intake throughout the day
- Evaluation of the severity of urinary incontinence
- Associated or provocative activities or events

patterns,[11] as there is poor correlation between subjective and charted estimates of diurnal and nocturnal urinary frequency.[12]

Pad test

The pad test is a simple, reliable, non-invasive test that quantifies loss by recording the weight change of the pad after it has been worn by the patient under investigation. More than 10 protocols have been described, which vary according to time and bladder filling.

The original evaluation of a one-hour pad test was published in 1981[13] and found that pad-weight change of more than 1 g should be regarded as abnormal and worthy of further investigation. In another study comparing continent and incontinent women, the 99% upper confidence limit for urine loss was 1.4 g in continent women with normal urodynamics.[14] The ICS has set the upper limit of normal for a one-hour pad test as 2 g.[15] The ICS standardized pad test[16] consists of drinking 500 ml of sodium-free liquid within a 15-minute time frame. A pre-weighed perineal pad is placed into the individual's underwear, following which a series of set manoeuvres are carried out, eg:

- coughing
- climbing stairs
- bending down.

The test is performed for one hour unless either the patient or investigator feel that it was not

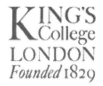

King's College Hospital London
Frequency Volume Chart

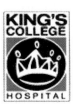

Time	Day 1			Day 2			Day 3		
	In	Out	Wet	In	Out	Wet	In	Out	Wet
7 am		340						260	
8 am	300			400	330		350		
9 am		200						170	
10 am	200	150		150	200		200		
11 am			W		175			150	
12 pm		200		150				50	
1 pm	150			150	200	W			
2 pm		175					320	200	
3 pm				200				200	
4 pm	450	150			220				W
5 pm		100					150		
6 pm		100	W	300			150	175	
7 pm	250	175		500	200 150				
8 pm	200	50		400	150 150	W	450	100	
9 pm	100				50	W		100	W
10 pm	350	180 BED		150			400	200	
11 pm					210 BED			210 BED	
12 am									
1 am		270					200		
2 am	100					W			
3 am		300							
4 am					210				
5 am									
6 am									

Figure 3.1
Frequency–volume chart

representative, in which case it may be continued for a further hour. The patient then voids, and the volume is recorded.

The short (one-hour) pad test is ideal because it is reproducible, easily administered and differentiates between continence and incontinence. It is less useful for objective quantification of urinary loss and has a significant false-negative rate. The long pad test (24–48 hours) is more cumbersome as it requires patients to collect, keep and return used pads. However, it has very high sensitivity and specificity, and is probably the most useful method for detection of incontinence where standard investigations have been normal.

> The long pad test lasts between 1 and 2 days, and although it is awkward (relying on patients to keep and return their used pads), it is a very sensitive method for detecting incontinence

Specialist investigations

Urodynamics

'Urodynamics' is a term used to describe a combination of tests that look at the ability of the bladder to store and expel urine.[17] It is most important to differentiate between symptoms and diagnoses (commonly by conventional laboratory urodynamics using artificial filling, or ambulatory urodynamics using physiological filling) whilst reproducing everyday activities. Symptoms of lower urinary tract dysfunction are often misleading. Studies have repeatedly shown the greater value of urodynamics over symptoms alone in diagnostic accuracy.[18, 19]

> Urodynamics is more useful and accurate for diagnosing lower urinary tract dysfunction than just symptoms alone

Uroflowmetry

It is easy to screen for the presence of voiding difficulty. This manifests as slow or incomplete micturition. Uroflowmetry plots the flow rate of urine over time and represents it graphically Figure 3.2 (a–d). Women should be encouraged to attend the hospital or clinic with a comfortably full bladder, so that they void for the test within their 'functional' range. Further investigation by pressure–flow analysis during cystometry discriminates between outflow obstruction (high pressure–low flow) and detrusor failure (low pressure–low flow).

> Uroflowmetry measures the flow rate of urine over time and plots it on a graph. It can be used to screen for voiding difficulty

Women attending hospital for urodynamics suffer high levels of anxiety, comparable to that of women attending gynaecology outpatient clinics.[20] Studies have previously

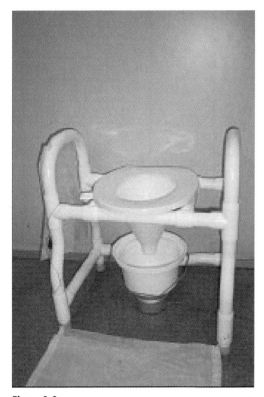

Figure 3.2a
Uroflowmeter

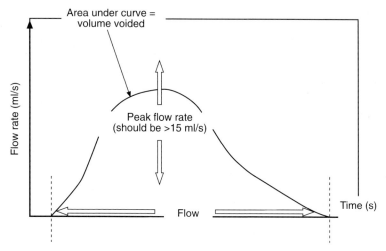

Figure 3.2b
Diagrammatic representation of normal urinary flow rate

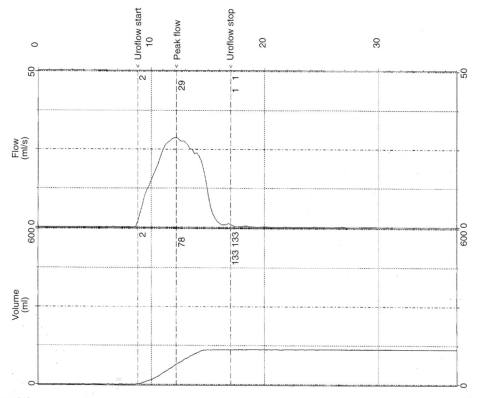

Figure 3.2c
Normal uroflowmetry study. The study shows the maximum flow rate (in this case 29ml/s) and the volume voided (in this case 133ml)

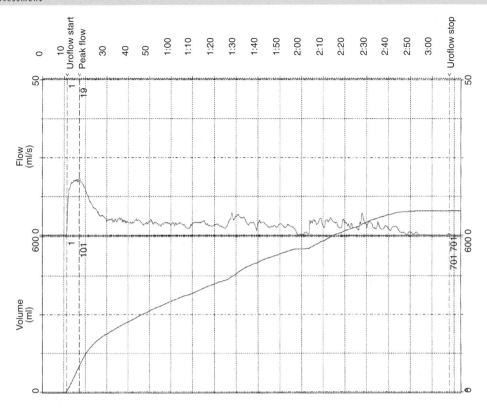

Figure 3.2d
Protracted uroflowmetry study. This study shows a good initial flow rate, but then a protracted void time

shown that only 2% of women sit directly on the seat in public toilets, whereas 85% crouch above the seat.[21] Approximately 38% of respondents crouch above the seat even in their friends' toilets! The same study demonstrated a 21% reduction in mean flow rate and 149% increase in residual volume in the crouching position. It is therefore essential that uroflowmetry be undertaken in private, preferably behind a locked door, and women should be specifically instructed to sit for the test.

> To make women comfortable and relaxed during the uroflowmetry test, they should be in a private, locked room and should be asked specifically to sit on the seat

Cystometry

When considering surgical treatment of UI it is important to be clear about the underlying cause. Whereas USI is often successfully treated by surgical intervention, DO is not. Indeed it may be made worse by incontinence surgery.

The technique of cystometry is well established. A filling catheter and fluid-filled pressure transducer are inserted into the bladder via the urethra. A fluid-filled pressure transducer is then inserted into the rectum via the anus or the vagina. Subtraction of the intraabdominal pressure from the intravesical pressure (subtraction cystometry) allows assessment of the relationship between pressure and volume during filling and of detrusor function by flowmetry during voiding. Single-channel (intravesical pressure) cystometry is equally sensitive but less specific, leading to over-diagnosis of DO (Figure 3.3a–d).

The catheters are inserted while the woman is in the supine position. The patient is then seated comfortably in the reclining/sitting position and the bladder is filled with saline, noting first sensation and capacity. Bladder filling is usually provocative – it is at a higher rate than the bladder would fill physiologically. Rates of filling vary from centre to centre, but are usually between 50 and 100 ml/minute, except in women with neurological disorders, for whom slow filling is employed.

During cystometry, the bladder is filled (through a catheter) with saline and the first sensations of filling, desire to void and bladder capacity are noted

The patient is asked to say when she first experiences a sensation of bladder filling. This usually occurs at 150–250 ml of fluid. This is followed by expression of the first desire to void, and strong desire to void. First desire to void usually occurs at 350–450 ml, and strong desire to void at maximum cystometric capacity, usually 400–600 ml of fluid. During filling, the patient is asked to cough at regular intervals to check subtraction, and to stand in order to

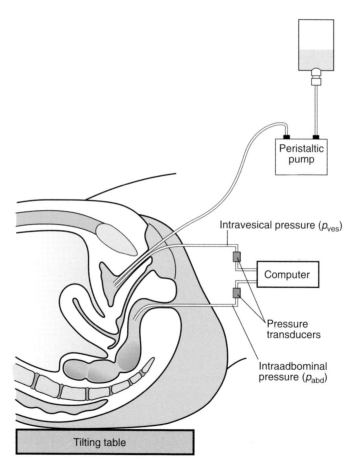

Figure 3.3a
Schematic drawing of catheter positions. Reprinted with permission from Cardozo L, Staskin D. *Textbook of Female Urology and Urogynaecology*. London: Taylor & Francis, 2001

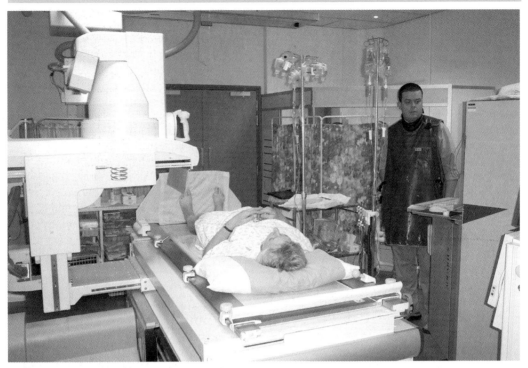

Figure 3.3b
Cystometry at King's College Hospital. Note the locked door and screens to ensure privacy for the women having urodynamics

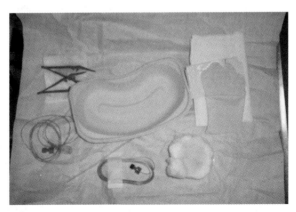

Figure 3.3c
Trolley set out for cystometry. Catheter and fluid-filled pressure transducers should be inserted using aseptic technique

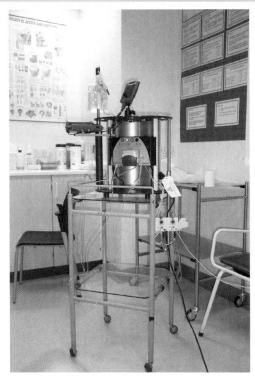 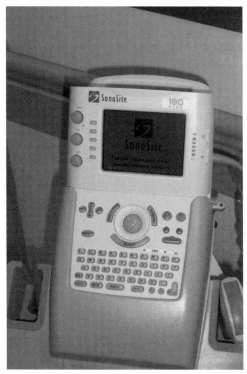

Figure 3.3d
Portable urodynamics. On the left is a Laborie Delphis portable urodynamics machine, incorporating uroflowmetry, subtracted cystometry and pressure–flow analysis. On the right is a Sonosite portable ultrasound machine as used at King's College Hospital

maximally provoke the bladder. The presence of detrusor contractions and leakage per urethram is noted – see Box 3.1.

Incontinence provoked by coughing in a patient with or without DO, but which occurs without an accompanying rise in detrusor pressure, is termed 'urethral sphincter incompetence' as opposed to USI. It is impossible to make any accurate assessment of the urethral sphincter when UI occurs in the presence of a rise in the detrusor pressure.

The patient is then asked to void at the end of the test, for pressure-flow analysis (Figure 3.4a–c).

Tests of urethral function

Tests of urethral function assess the closure pressure of the urethra, and thus the ability of the urethra to prevent leakage. If the closure or squeeze pressure of the urethra exceeds the intravesical pressure, then the woman should remain continent. Measurement may occur:

- over a period of time at one point in the urethra (continuous urethral pressure recording)
- at a single time along its length (urethral pressure profile).

Urethral closure pressure

Urethral pressure measurements have never been shown to be a useful discriminant of USI when used in isolation. Maximal urethral closure pressures decline with age and may be statistically lower in patients with USI. However, a single isolated assessment of urethral closure pressure carries no prognostic significance for a

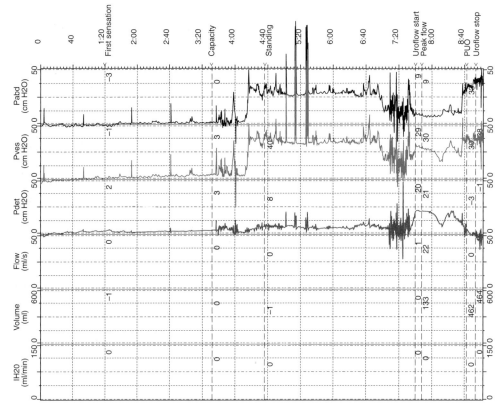

Figure 3.4a
Normal subtracted cystometry trace. Intravesical pressure (blue line) and abdominal pressure (black line) can be measured directly with transducers. Pdet (Detrusor Pressure) = Pves – Pabd. This is calculated continuously by the computer and plotted as the red line (Pdet). During this test there is no change in detrusor pressure despite provocation with coughing, standing and listening to running water. A normal pressure–flow analysis of voiding is also included at the end of the test

single individual. Urethral pressure profilometry has been shown to have a low reproducibility for both inter- and intra-observer testing,[22] largely because of normal biological changes in the urethra related to muscle tone. There is also little consensus on how the measurement should be taken or used, which further affects research and development of a useful clinical tool.

> Maximal urethral closure pressure usually declines with age and may also be lower in patients with USI

Leak-point pressure

Leak-point pressure provides limited information about the integrity and function of the urethral sphincter mechanism during the storage phase of the micturition cycle. However, it must be measured at a standard volume of 200 ml,[23] and the detrusor compliance must be normal. Bladder volume has a significant effect on leak-point pressure, with diminishing values as the bladder volume increases.

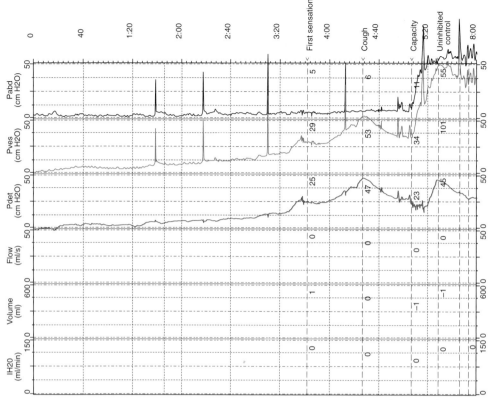

Figure 3.4b
Detrusor overactivity – systolic detrusor contractions are seen as the bladder approaches capacity. A provoked detrusor contraction is also seen on standing

Prolapse

Prolapse may 'mask' incontinence. Repair of prolapse may unmask pre-existing incontinence.[24] Therefore, the presence of leakage despite major prolapse implies severe urethral sphincter dysfunction.

Surgery

Tests of urethral function, whilst being of limited value in isolation, do confer some information about surgical success and prognosis. Intrinsic sphincter deficiency (ISD) preoperatively carries an increased risk of surgical failure.[25]

Video-urodynamics (videocystourethrography)

Video-urodynamics combines fluoroscopic imaging

of the bladder neck with cystometry by filling the bladder with iodine-based contrast medium. This allows differentiation between USI due to bladder neck hypermobility and that due to ISD. In addition, anatomical variants can be identified.

> Video-urodynamics combines fluoroscopic imaging of the bladder neck with cystometry. This is done by filling the bladder with iodine-based contrast medium

Video-urodynamics may also be used in the diagnosis of DO. Although the diagnosis is made primarily on an abnormal rise in detrusor pressure in combination with the patient's symptoms, a significant rise in intravesical pressure may lead to vesico-ureteric reflux and

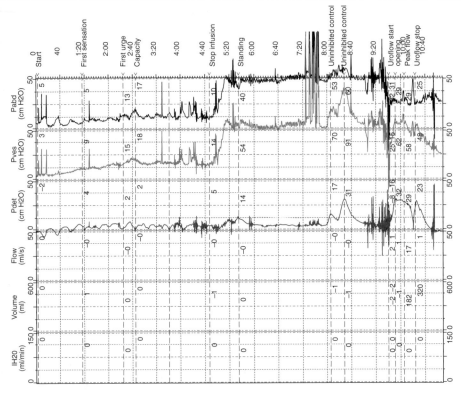

Figure 3.4c

Subtraction artefact should not be confused with detrusor contractions. Rectal peristalsis causes negative deflections on P_{det}, as the computer runs a continuous subtraction. Provoked detrusor contractions are seen later in the test after coughing

subsequent renal damage. This is especially common in women with neurogenic bladder problems. It is therefore important to be aware of any abnormalities in the renal tract, and the presence of vesico-ureteric reflux. This may be visualized by radiological screening during cystometry in either the filling or voiding phase.

Patients with spinal cord injury commonly suffer with lower urinary tract symptoms. Video-urodynamics is especially useful to detect detrusor–sphincter dyssynergia, where voiding difficulties are caused by failure of the urethral sphincter to relax at the same time as the detrusor muscle contracts (Figure 3.5a,b).

> Video-urodynamics is especially useful in detecting detrusor–sphincter dyssynergia

Ambulatory urodynamics

Recently ambulatory urodynamics has been used in the diagnosis of DO.[26] For this test, an intravesical and intrarectal pressure line is inserted (as for laboratory urodynamics) but no filling catheter is used. The bladder fills naturally with urine from the kidneys. A small recording device, similar in principle to a 24-hour ECG or blood pressure monitor, is worn, and the information is later downloaded to a computer for review.

This test is thought to be physiological, as non-provocative filling is used, and during the period of the test the woman should go about 'normal' activities (Figure 3.6), perhaps including those that cause her to be incontinent. The presence of pressure transducers in the bladder and urethra is uncomfortable and may be provocative, reducing the specificity of the test. It is thought to be a more sensitive test than laboratory urodynamics, detecting an extra 30% of cases of DO. The recordings of ambulatory urodynamics are analysed in the same way, with attention being directed at the correlation between pressure recordings and symptoms.

Imaging of the urinary tract

Imaging techniques used to look at the urinary tract include:

- ultrasonography
- micturating cystography
- intravenous urography
- magnetic resonance imaging
- cysto-urethroscopy

Ultrasonography

Ultrasonography of the urinary tract may be performed (Figure 3.7a,b). This can be useful to visualize the upper tracts when looking for dilatation secondary to reflux, or to estimate bladder capacity or post-void residual. More recently, bladder wall thickness has been used to assess the probability of DO – a thickened hypertrophied detrusor being associated with abnormal detrusor activity.[27]

Ultrasound is a rapid, painless method of examining the pelvis and abdomen, and reveals a high number of incidental ultrasound findings, such as ovarian cysts or uterine fibroids. This is true regardless of the source of referral.[28] Such space-occupying lesions may profoundly affect lower urinary tract function. Ultrasound cannot yet, however, replace tests of dynamic function.

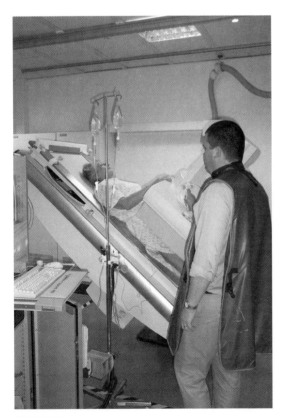
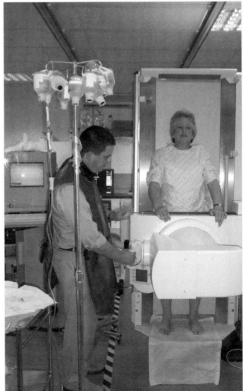

Figure 3.5a
Provocation by standing and coughing during video-urodynamics

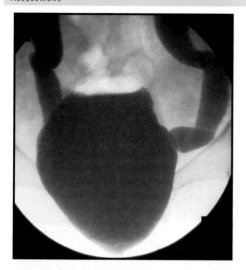

Figure 3.5b
Ureteric reflux. This series of scans demonstrates severe bilateral ureteric reflux, causing distension and blunting of the renal pelvic calyces, as seen during video-urodynamics. They were associated with DO in this woman. It is vital to make the diagnosis, to identify possible current or future risk of renal damage.

Micturating cystography

In isolation, a micturating cystogram is useful to diagnose fistulae and diverticula (Figure 3.8a,b). It is more useful to combine it with dual-channel subtracted cystometry at video-urodynamics.

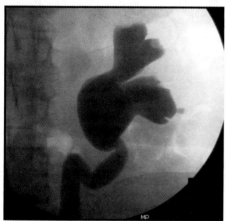

Intravenous urography/intravenous pyelography

An intravenous urograph is useful for imaging the upper renal tracts (Figure 3.9), and is often used in conjunction with ultrasound to investigate:

- recurrent UTI
- recurrent haematuria
- outflow obstruction
- known cases of vesico-ureteric reflux.

Ureteric fistulae and filling defects (associated with pathology such as transitional cell carcinoma and calculus) may also be detected.

Magnetic resonance imaging

Magnetic resonance imaging (MRI) has improved the anatomical investigation of incontinence and prolapse because of the highly detailed images now available. Specifically, understanding of the normal pelvic anatomy and comparative studies after childbirth has advanced our knowledge of the mechanisms of incontinence and prolapse.[29] In the UK MRI remains predominantly a research (and tertiary centre) investigative technique because of cost and availability.

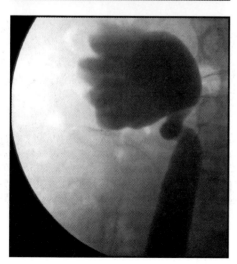

> MRI is mainly a research/investigative technique in the UK because of its cost and availability

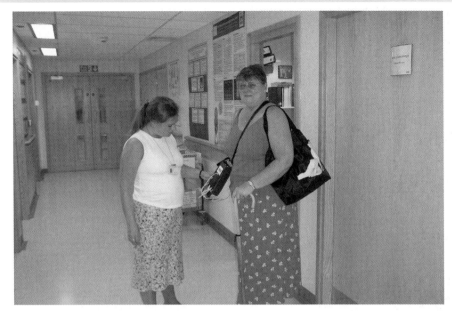

Figure 3.6
Ambulatory urodynamics

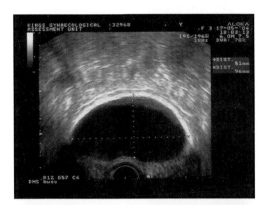

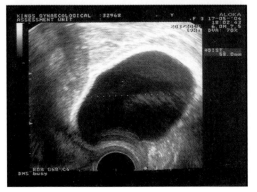

Figure 3.7a
Ultrasound estimation of post-void residual. The bladder volume in millilitres is given by the formula: (Height cm × Width cm × Depth cm) × 0.7

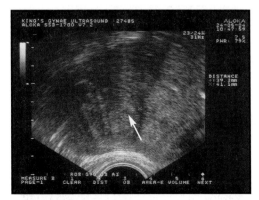

Figure 3.7b
Uterine fibroid as an incidental finding. Fibroids, often clinically suspected or an incidental finding, can cause pressure symptoms on the bladder.

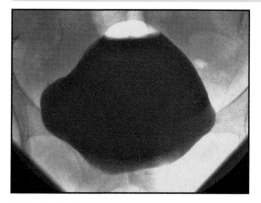

Figure 3.8a
The normal bladder outline. This is the bladder as seen at micturating cystogram or video-urodynamics. The bladder neck is well supported in an intraabdominal position

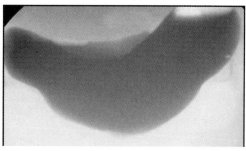

Figure 3.8b
Bladder distorted by fibroids. Although this bladder neck is also well supported, the outline of the bladder is markedly distorted by fibroid compression. (The diagnosis should be confirmed by ultrasound to exclude a large ovarian cyst.)

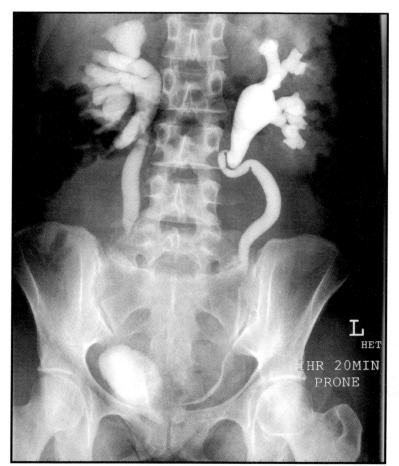

Figure 3.9
Intravenous urography/intravenous pyelography (IVP) This IVP was taken to investigate a woman who attended our urogynaecology outpatients clinic with urgency/frequency symptoms. She was noted to have a huge fibroid uterus, which is compressing her ureters, causing bilateral hydronephrosis. GnRH analogue was administered, and urgent abdominal hysterectomy was advised

Cysto-urethroscopy

It is not necessary for all women to undergo cystoscopy (Figure 3.10), but it may be useful in selected cases, eg:

- sensory urgency
- unexplained/persistent haematuria (especially in women aged over 40 years)
- failure to respond to conventional treatment
- bladder pain.

When DO is secondary to bladder stones or malignancy, this is revealed at the time of cysto-urethroscopy.

Conclusion

The appropriate investigation of lower urinary tract symptoms is of paramount importance in order to secure an accurate diagnosis. Urinary symptoms alone are not sufficient to gain an accurate impression of the underlying pathology, and this may lead to inappropriate treatment being given and deterioration of the patient's condition and quality of life.

For an overview of the management strategy used at King's College Hospital to investigate

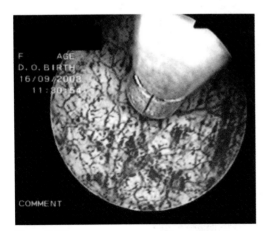

Figure 3.10
Cystoscopy reveals abnormal petechial haemorrhage in investigation of bladder pain. The biopsy forceps are seen in the centre of the picture. Biopsy is useful to obtain a histological diagnosis and exclude malignancy

uro-genital dysfunction, please refer to the inside front cover.

References

1. Sand PK, Hill RC, Ostergard DR. Incontinence history as a predictor for detrusor instability. *Obstet Gynecol* 1988; **71**: 257–9.

2. Abrams P, Cardozo L, Fall M *et al.* The standardisation of terminology in lower urinary tract function. *Neurourol Urodyn* 2002; **21**: 167–78.

3. Cutner A, Cardozo LD, Benness CJ. Assessment of urinary symptoms in early pregnancy. *Br J Obstet Gynaecol* 1991; **98**: 1283–6.

4. Cutner A, Cardozo LD, Benness CJ. Assessment of urinary symptoms in the second half of pregnancy. *Int Urogynaecol J* 1992; **3**: 30–2.

5. Bump RC, Mattiasson A, Bo K *et al.* The standardisation of terminology of female pelvic organ prolapse and pelvic floor dysfunction. *Am J Obstet Gynecol* 1996; **175**: 10–11.

6. World Health Organization. *Definition of Health from Preamble to the Constitution of the WHO Basic Documents, 28th edition.* Geneva: WHO, 1978.

7. Naughton MJ, Shumaker SA. Assessment of health related quality of life. In: Furberg CD, DeMets DL (eds). *Fundamentals of Clinical Trials, 3rd edition.* St Louis: Mosby, 1996, p 185.

8. Gill TM, Feinstein AR. A critical appraisal of the quality of life measurements. *JAMA* 1974; **272**: 619–26.

9. Kass EH. Bacteruria and the diagnosis of infections of the lower urinary tract. *AMA Arch Int Med* 1957; **100**: 709–14.

10. Abrams P, Fenely R, Torrens M. Patient Assessment. In Abrams P, Fenely R, Torrens M (eds). *Urodynamics, 1st edition.* New York: Springer, 1983, pp 6–27.

11. Larsson G, Victor A. Micturition patterns in a healthy female population, studied with a frequency–volume chart. *Scand J Urol Nephrol Suppl* 1988; **114**: 53–7.

12. McCormack M, Infante-Rivard C, Schick E. Agreement between clinical methods of measurement of urinary frequency and functional bladder capacity. *Br J Urol* 1992; **9**: 17–21.

13. Sutherst J, Brown M, Shawer M. Assessing the severity of urinary incontinence in women by weighing perineal pads. *Lancet* 1981; **i**: 1128–30.

14. Versi E, Cardozo L. Perineal pad weighing versus videographic analysis in genuine stress incontinence. *Br J Obstet Gynaecol* 1986; **93**: 364–6.

15. Abrams P, Blaivas JG, Stanton SL *et al.* The standardization of terminology of lower urinary tract function. *Scand J Urol Nephrol Suppl* 1988; **114**: 5–19.

16. Abrams P, Blaivas JG, Stanton SL, Andersen JT. The standardisation of terminology of lower urinary tract function. *Neurourol Urodyn* 1988; **7**: 403–26.

17. Hosker G. ICS (UK) Annual Scientific Meeting, Leicester. 24-25 April 2003. Expert presentation.

18. Jarvis GJ, Hall S, Stamp S, Millar DR. An assessment of urodynamic investigation in incontinent women. *Br J Obstet Gynaecol* 1980; **87**: 873–96.

19. James M, Jackson S, Shepherd A, Abrams P. Pure stress leakage symptomatology: Is it safe to discount detrusor instability? *Br J Obstet Gynaecol* 1999; **106**: 1255–8.

20. Parsons M, Williams M, Cardozo L. Anxiety during urodynamics. *Int Urogynaecol J* 2003 [Proceedings of the 28th Annual Meeting of the International Urogynaecology Association, Buenos Aires (Supplement S10)].

21. Moore KH, Richmond DH, Sutherst JR *et al*. Crouching over the toilet seat: prevalence among British gynaecological outpatients and its effect upon micturition. *Br J Obstet Gynaecol* 1991; **98**: 569–72.

22. Lose G. Urethral pressure measurements. In Staskin D, Cardozo LD (eds). *Textbook of Female Urology and Urogynaecology*. Oxford: Isis Medical Media 2001, pp 215–26.

23. Haab F, Dmochowski R, Zimmern P, Leach GE. The variability of the leakage pressure threshold due to exertion 'the Valsalva Leak Point Pressure' as a function of the filling volume of the bladder. *Prog Urol* 1997; **7**: 422–5.

24. Hextall A, Boos K, Cardozo L *et al*. Videocystourethrography with a ring pessary in situ. A clinically useful preoperative investigation for continent women with urogenital prolapse? *Int Urogynecol J Pelvic Floor Dysfunct* 1998; **9**: 205–9.

25. Francis LN, Sand PK, Hamrang K, Ostergard DR. A urodynamic appraisal of success and failure after retropubic urethropexy. *J Reprod Med* 1987; **32**: 693–6.

26. van Waalwijk van Doorn ES, Zwiers W, Wetzels LL, Debruyne FM. A comparative study between standard and ambulant urodynamics. *Neurourol Urodyn* 1987; **6**: 156.

27. Khullar V, Salvatore S, Cardozo LD *et al*. Ultrasound bladder wall measurement – a non-invasive screening test for detrusor instability. *Neurourol Urodyn* 1994; **13**: 461–2.

28. Mills P, Joseph AE, Adam EJ. Total abdominal and pelvic ultrasound: incidental findings and a comparison between outpatient and general practice referrals in 1000 cases. *Br J Radiol* 1989; **62**: 974–6.

29. DeLancey JO, Kearney R, Chou Q *et al*. The appearance of levator ani muscle abnormalities in magnetic resonance images after vaginal delivery. *Obstet Gynecol* 2003; **101**: 46–53.

4. Classification

Causes of incontinence
Classification of incontinence
Other factors
Conclusion

The lower urinary tract consists of two synergistic components:

- the bladder, to store and void
- the urethra, to control and convey.

The relationship between these two organs is under complex neurological control and is the basis of normal lower urinary tract function, and therefore continence. Lower urinary tract symptoms 'are the subjective indicator of a disease or change in condition as perceived by the patient, carer or partner and may lead him/her to seek help from the healthcare professional'.[1]

The International Continence Society (ICS) classifies lower urinary tract dysfunction into disorders of the storage and voiding phases of the micturition cycle.[1, 2] Adequate cognitive function, mobility, motivation and manual dexterity provide the means to perform the tasks of continence. It follows, therefore, that disruption of any of these functions can lead to incontinence.[3] Assuming the absence of inflammation, infection or neoplasm, lower urinary tract dysfunction can be caused by:

- disturbances of neurological or psychological control
- disorders of muscle function
- structural abnormalities.

> Lower urinary tract dysfunction can be caused by structural abnormalities, disturbances of neurological or psychological control, or disorders of muscle function

Causes of incontinence

The major causes of chronic incontinence, therefore, can be summarized as

- urodynamic stress incontinence – previously known as 'genuine stress incontinence'
- detrusor overactivity – previously known as 'detrusor instability'
- overflow incontinence
- functional incontinence
- transient/acute incontinence
- fistula
- congenital abnormality
- urethral diverticulum.

Urodynamic stress incontinence (USI), detrusor overactivity (DO), mixed incontinence and overflow incontinence are by far the commonest causes of incontinence in the UK. Urodynamic stress incontinence accounts for approximately 50% of cases, DO for around 40% and overflow for most of the remaining 10%. Many women present with 'mixed incontinence', which is usually a combination of stress urinary incontinence with DO.

> The most common causes of incontinence in the UK are USI (50%), DO (40%), mixed incontinence and overflow incontinence

Fistulae

Fistulae are rare in England and are usually secondary to gynaecological surgery, malignancy or radiotherapy. A fistula is an abnormal connection between two epithelial surfaces. Surgical procedures associated with vesicovaginal fistulae include:

- total abdominal hysterectomy
- vaginal hysterectomy
- anterior repair
- radical hysterectomy
- laparoscopic pelvic surgery
- urological procedures.

In addition, damage to the bladder following pelvic radiotherapy has also been associated with vesicovaginal fistulae. Mechanisms involved in the causation of fistulae include:

- anatomical distortion by fibroids or endometriosis
- failure to recognize and repair direct bladder damage
- inappropriate suture placement.

Obstetric fistulae are much commoner in the developing world and are a frequent reason why women are cast out of their homes and communities and abandoned.

Urethrovaginal and ureterovaginal fistulae are much less common than vesicovaginal fistulae. In the developed world they are unusual causes of urinary incontinence (UI). Once again, the most common cause of these fistuale in the developing world is obstetric trauma due to ischaemic necrosis; in developed countries the most common cause is surgery. Anterior repair, vaginal hysterectomy and urethral diverticulectomy have all been associated with an increased risk of urethral fistula formation. Congenital causes of UI include:

- ectopic ureter
- epispadias
- bladder exstrophy
- cloacal exstrophy.

Classification of urinary incontinence

Urodynamic stress incontinence

USI, as opposed to the patient symptom 'stress urinary incontinence' (SUI), is only diagnosed after performing urodynamics and is the involuntary leakage of urine per urethram during periods of raised intraabdominal pressure, in the absence of a detrusor contraction.

> USI is the involuntary leakage of urine during periods of raised intraabdominal pressure in the absence of detrusor contractions

Normal urethral function maintains a positive urethral closure pressure in the presence of raised intraabdominal pressure, although DO may overcome it. An incompetent urethra allows leakage of urine, even in the absence of a detrusor contraction. Damage to the pubo-urethral ligaments and the levator ani muscles (secondary to pregnancy, childbirth, obesity, radical pelvic surgery, abdominopelvic mass or chronic cough, and possibly exacerbated by inherited weak collagen) may allow bladder-neck hypermobility and descent of the bladder neck and proximal urethra, so that they are no longer within the intraabdominal pressure zone.

Intrinsic damage to the rhabdosphincter or a scarred drainpipe urethra that cannot occlude properly[4] may occur after:

- vaginal surgery
- previous incontinence surgery
- urethral dilatation, chronic urethritis
- radiotherapy.

Electromyographic studies have demonstrated denervation of the intrinsic and extrinsic sphincter mechanisms.[5,6] This is known as 'intrinsic sphincter deficiency', where the hermetic closure properties of the proximal urethra are lost and USI may be the result.

Treatment

The mainstays of treatment for USI in the UK are:

- conservative management with containment aids
- treatment with physiotherapy
- recourse to surgery where indicated and desired.

From September 2004 the first drug treatment for SUI, duloxetine, will be available. It is essential to be sure of the diagnosis by excluding DO (see Chapter 6) – a minority of patients opting for a surgical treatment develop irritative symptoms of urgency and frequency or voiding difficulty postoperatively, and pre-existing symptoms are likely to be exacerbated.

Before treating USI or SUI it is important to exclude DO

Detrusor overactivity

DO is a urodynamic observation characterized by involuntary detrusor contractions that may be spontaneous or provoked. The contractions occur during the filling phase. *Phasic DO* is defined by a characteristic waveform that mimics the normal voiding cycle, but which does not inevitably lead to UI. *Terminal DO* is defined as a single involuntary detrusor contraction at cystometric capacity, which cannot be suppressed, and leads to incontinence – usually complete – and catastrophic bladder emptying.[7] *Provoked DO* is the association of a detrusor contraction with either a physical provocation to the bladder, such as coughing and standing, or a psychological provocation such as hearing running water.

DO is an urodynamic observation characterized by involuntary detrusor contractions that may be spontaneous or provoked

Low compliance

Alternatively, the bladder may demonstrate *low compliance*, possibly as a separate entity or possibly as an end-stage phenomenon and characterized by an abnormal rise in the detrusor pressure during filling. There are a variety of causes, including:

- radiotherapy
- radical pelvic surgery
- recurrent urinary tract infection (UTI)
- extrinsic mass causing pressure
- interstitial cystitis.

Symptomatically, these patients are similar to, and often indistinguishable from, patients with DO. Sometimes, however, low compliance may be associated with a fast bladder-filling rate. Low compliance is seen less often at

physiological filling rates (eg in ambulatory studies).[1]

Patients with DO are often indistinguishable from patients with low compliance; however, low compliance may be associated with a fast bladder-filling rate and is seen less often at physiological filling rates

Pathophysiology and idiopathic DO

The incidence of DO increases with age, and urge incontinence is the commonest symptom of incontinence in people aged over 60 years[8] and the elderly.[9] Urodynamic assessment is required to make an accurate diagnosis, as women usually present with multiple symptoms, most commonly a syndrome of frequency, urgency and nocturia. The pathophysiology of DO is poorly understood and an underlying cause is rarely found, leading to the term *idiopathic DO*. Detrusor overactivity and USI can coexist as mixed incontinence and DO can arise *de novo* after incontinence surgery.

The process of toilet training in young children is the learning of cortical inhibition of detrusor contractions. Many researchers feel that idiopathic DO is either an 'unlearning' or poor initial learning of this control. There is also evidence that idiopathic DO is caused by a functional denervation injury of the detrusor muscle.[10]

It is thought that idiopathic DO may be an 'unlearning' of cortical inhibition of detrusor contractions, ie toilet training, or is due to a functional denervation injury of the detrusor muscle

Any neurological lesion or condition that interrupts the cortical inhibition of detrusor contractions can result in *neurogenic DO*, eg multiple sclerosis or spinal cord lesions. Urethral outflow obstruction can lead to incomplete bladder emptying, and subsequent symptoms of urgency and frequency.

Treatment

Treatment consists of a combination of bladder retraining and 'bladder drill', with anticholinergic medication to help relearn the cortical inhibition of detrusor contractions. This may be time-consuming and frustrating – correct diagnosis is necessary to ensure maximum patient compliance with this treatment.

Overflow incontinence

Overflow incontinence occurs when the bladder, secondary to an injury or insult, becomes large and flaccid, and has little or no detrusor tone or function. The condition is diagnosed when the urinary residual is more than 50% of the capacity. The bladder simply leaks as it becomes full – the sequelae of this are:

- reduced functional capacity
- increased frequency of micturition
- recurrent urinary tract infection.

In the longer term, there may be hydroureter, hydronephrosis, and chronic renal failure secondary to reflux nephropathy.

> Patients with overflow incontinence may go on to develop hydroureter, hydronephrosis or chronic renal failure in the long term

These injuries can occur because of injudicious and inappropriate care of the bladder after epidural anaesthesia. In the obstetric setting, lack of sensation or awareness in the mother, in combination with a busy postnatal ward, may mean that the mother does not pass urine for many hours after leaving the delivery suite. Inappropriate management, combined with a post-partum diuresis, can result in several overdistension injuries, compounding the original problem. Even a single episode of overdistension may result in permanently impaired detrusor function. The female bladder is especially sensitive to overdistension – the causes are several-fold, and are set out in Table 4.1.

Table 4.1
Common causes of overflow incontinence.
Overflow incontinence can be caused by a variety of insults that may impair the ability of the bladder to empty appropriately. The commonest causes are listed here

Insult	Example
Acute retention	• Secondary to surgery, especially gynaecological and rectal
	• Pain, eg herpes simplex, shingles
Drugs	• Tricyclic antidepressants
	• Anticholinergics
	• Diuretics
	• α-agonists
	• Epidural anaesthesia
Urinary tract infection	
Urethral stricture	• Surgery for urodynamic stress incontinence
	• Urethral surgery, especially dilatations
	• Vaginal surgery
Pelvic mass	• Fibroid uterus
	• Faecal impaction
Cystocele	
Detrusor failure	• Lower motor neurone lesion, eg diabetic neuropathy
	• Overdistension injury
Psychogenic	• Dementia

> Overdistension may result in permanent impairment of detrusor function

Functional and transient incontinence

Functional incontinence includes cases of UI where no organic cause can be found. Several other factors may be responsible for problems with incontinence due to interference with voiding behaviour. These include cognitive factors, such as dementia and learning difficulties, as well as physical factors, such as immobility and disability.

Untreated acute incontinence is likely to become persistent, but is not considered

Delirium

Infection

Atrophic change

Pharmacological

Psychological

Excess urine output

Restricted mobility

Stool impaction

Figure 4.1
The mnemonic DIAPPERS

chronic simply because it is long-standing. These causes have been summarized by the mnemonic 'DIAPPERS', see Figure 4.1.[11]

Acute incontinence

Symptomatic UTI is a cause of acute incontinence, especially in young women, often because of extreme frequency, urgency and pain. If symptoms persist, despite negative cultures, it is worth considering culture for fastidious organisms, such as *Chlamydia trachomatis*, *Ureaplasma urealyticum* or *Mycoplasma hominis*. Alternatively, empirical treatment might be considered. Atrophic urethritis and/or vaginitis in postmenopausal women are often associated with urinary tract symptoms. These conditions are due to epithelial and submucosal thinning of the urethra, with consequential irritation and loss of the mucosal seal. Incontinence associated with atrophic urethritis tends to be characterized by urgency and occasionally 'scalding' dysuria, and may be underreported.[12] Treatment with local oestrogen cream or hormone replacement therapy is as effective as oral therapy in correcting atrophy.[13]

> Atrophy can be corrected using local application of oestrogen cream or hormone replacement therapy

Alcohol and medications are major causes of acute incontinence in the elderly. Polypharmacy

and the use of psychotropic medication compound problems with incontinence, and are most prevalent in women aged 85 years or over. The prevalence appears to be increasing (Table 4.2).[14]

Other factors

Excessive urine output is caused by:

- high fluid intake
- diuretic use (including caffeine and alcohol)
- metabolic abnormalities, most typically hyperglycaemia or hypercalcaemia.

Nighttime incontinence can be exacerbated by return of peripheral oedema fluid in heart failure, peripheral venous insufficiency and hypoalbuminaemia.

Other reasons for UI include cognitive impairment, such as dementia, as well as physical immobility and disability, and these may be responsible for exacerbating the impact of incontinence.

> Urinary incontinence can be caused by:
> - high fluid intake
> - diuretic use
> - cognitive impairment
> - physical immobility
> - metabolic abnormalities (eg hyperglycaemia or hypercalcaemia)

Restricted mobility may alter the balance between coping and not coping with lower urinary tract symptoms, simply by limiting the ability of an individual to reach the toilet in time. It may be a result of physical limitation of age, by a medical condition confining her to bed or to a chair, or from subtle and correctable factors, such as:

- poorly fitting shoes
- failing vision or altered optical prescription
- postural hypotension
- fear of falling on steep stairs or loose carpets.

Table 4.2

Drugs that may aggravate or predispose to urinary incontinence. An increasing trend towards polypharmacy in the elderly exacerbates the problems of the effects of drugs on the lower urinary tract

Class of drug	Examples	Unwanted effects
Alcohol		Polyuria, frequency, urgency, sedation, delirium, immobility
Diuretics	Furosemide, caffeine	Polyuria, frequency, urgency
Anticholinergics	Antihistamine	Urinary retention and overflow, delirium, faecal impaction
Antidepressants (tricyclic)	Amitriptyline, imipramine	Anticholinergic actions, sedation
Antipsychotics	Haloperidol, thioridazine	Anticholinergic actions, sedation, rigidity, immobility
Sedatives/hypnotics	Diazepam	Sedation, delirium, immobility
Narcotic analgesia delirium	Opioids	Urinary retention, faecal impaction, sedation,
α-blockers	Prazosin, doxazosin	Urethral relaxation and stress incontinence (in women)
Calcium-channel blockers	Nifedipine, diltiazem	Decreased detrusor contractility, urinary retention, nocturia from peripheral oedema, impaction
Prostaglandins	Misoprostol	Urethral relaxation, stress incontinence
Angiotensin-converting enzyme (ACE) inhibitors	Captopril, enalapril	Cough (may precipitate or worsen stress leakage)
NSAIDs	Diclofenac, ibuprofen	Salt and water retention
H$_2$ antagonists	Ranitidine, cimetidine	Confusion

A simple urinal or bedside commode may resolve the problem.

Stool impaction (constipation) causes urinary incontinence, especially in elderly patients and children. Typical presentations are symptoms of urgency or overflow incontinence, and associated faecal incontinence. Removing the impacted stool may restore continence. Additionally, constipation and straining at stool, as a young adult, are risk factors for the development of prolapse and stress incontinence in later life.[15]

> Constipation and straining at stool when young are risk factors for developing prolapse and incontinence later in life

Conclusion

The investigation and treatment of lower urinary tract dysfunction and UI is an increasingly complex and specialized area of medical expertise. The high prevalence in the community, in combination with a reluctance to seek help, or perhaps the feeling that incontinence is an expected normal part of ageing, mean that there is a large cohort of women who remain undiagnosed. In the past the classification system used has varied between countries, making communication and cooperation with regard to treatment and research complicated. However, the ICS has published consensus documents to standardize nomenclature and investigation.

The commonest cause of UI in the UK remains USI, with DO the second highest cause. Together they account for around 90% of all diagnoses, with overflow incontinence making up most of the rest. Fistulae and congenital abnormalities remain very rare. It is important to distinguish adequately between USI and DO by laboratory or ambulatory urodynamics, as necessary, prior to considering surgical treatment.

There are some transient, or acute, causes of incontinence that are particularly important in the elderly because appropriate treatment of the underlying cause may effectively treat the incontinence. Medical and surgical conditions and side-effects of ongoing treatments may initiate or exacerbate lower urinary tract symptoms. They may become persistent if not treated promptly.

References

1. Abrams P, Cardozo L, Fall M et al. The standardisation of terminology of lower urinary tract function: report from the Standardisation Sub-Committee of the International Continence Society. Neurourol Urodyn 2002; 21: 167–78.

2. Abrams P, Blaivas JG, Stanton S, Andersen JT. The standardisation of terminology of lower urinary tract function. Neurourol Urodyn 1988; 7: 403–26.

3. Beers M, Berkow R (eds). Urinary incontinence. In: The Merck Manual of Diagnosis and Therapy, 17th edition (Centennial Edition), Section 17. Merck publications.

4. Keller C. Epidemiology and classification of incontinence. In: Cardozo LD (ed). Urogynaecology. Edinburgh: Churchill Livingstone 1997, pp 3–23.

5. Smith AR, Hosker GL, Warrell DW. The role of pudendal nerve damage in the aetiology of genuine stress incontinence in women. Br J Obstet Gynaecol 1989; 96: 29–32.

6. Allen RE, Hosker GL, Smith AR, Warrell DW. Pelvic floor damage and childbirth: a neurophysiological study. Br J Obstet Gynaecol 1990; 97: 770–9.

7. Monga A. Incontinence in women: an overview. In: MacLean A, Cardozo L (eds). Incontinence in Women. London: RCOG Press, 2002, pp 3–13.

8. Brown JS. OAB: Broadening our understanding and impact. Key Issues in the Treatment of Overactive Bladder. Seminar Session, 32nd Annual Meeting of the ICS, 2002.

9. Castleden CM, Duffin HM, Asher MJ. Clinical and urodynamic studies in 100 elderly patients. Br Med J Clin Res 1981; 282: 1103–5.

10. Brading AF, Turner WH. The unstable bladder: towards a common mechanism. Br J Urol 1994; 73: 3–8.

11. Resnick NM, Yalla SV. Current concepts: management of urinary incontinence in the elderly. N Engl J Med 1985; 313: 800–15.

12. Hextall A, Cardozo L. Managing postmenopausal cystitis. Hosp Pract 1997; 32: 191–8.

13. Cardozo L, Bachmann G, McClish D et al. Meta-analysis of estrogen therapy in the management of uro-genital atrophy in post-menopausal women: second report of the Hormones and Urogenital Therapy Committee. Obstet Gynecol 1998; 92(4 Pt 2): 722–7.

14. Linjakumpu T, Hartikainen S, Klaukka T et al. Psychotropics among the home-dwelling elderly – increasing trends. Int J Geriatr Psych 2002; 17: 874–83.

15. Spence-Jones C, Kamm MA, Henry MM, Hudson CN. Bowel dysfunction: a pathogenic factor in utero-vaginal prolapse and urinary stress incontinence. Br J Obstet Gynaecol 1994; 101: 147–52.

5. Urodynamic stress incontinence

Introduction
Definition
Pathophysiology and aetiology
Clinical features
Investigations
Treatment
Summary

Introduction

Urodynamic stress incontinence (USI) is the commonest cause of urinary incontinence in the UK. It represents around 50% of all diagnoses. An epidemiological survey of 29 500 households across four European countries also showed that stress incontinence is the commonest presenting symptom, with 42% of respondents admitting to stress-type incontinence in the preceding 30 days.[1]

Definition

Urodynamic stress incontinence (as opposed to the patient symptom 'stress incontinence') is only diagnosed after performing urodynamics, and is the involuntary leakage of urine per urethram during periods of raised intraabdominal pressure, in the absence of a detrusor contraction.[2]

> Urodynamic stress incontinence can only be diagnosed after performing urodynamics

Pathophysiology and aetiology

Normal urethral function maintains a positive urethral closure pressure in the presence of raised intraabdominal pressure, although detrusor overactivity (DO) may overcome it. An incompetent urethra allows leakage of urine, even in the absence of a detrusor contraction. In 1976 Enhorning described the theory of simultaneous transmission of pressure to the proximal urethra,[3] which he maintained was held above the level of the pelvic floor in continent women.

Damage to the pubo-urethral ligaments and the levator ani muscles – possibly secondary to pregnancy, childbirth, obesity, radical pelvic surgery, abdominopelvic mass or chronic cough – may allow bladder-neck hypermobility and descent of the bladder neck and proximal urethra, so that they are no longer within the intraabdominal pressure zone. Greenwald, however, caused doubt by demonstrating a lack of correlation between intraabdominal position of the bladder neck and stress incontinence.[4] A rise in urethral pressure prior to coughing would suggest a reflex action, which would not be supported by Enhorning's theory.[5]

The 'Integral Theory' is based on experimental and clinical studies describing the anatomy and function of the female pelvic floor and the urethral closure mechanism. The central theme of the theory is that the vagina acts as a 'hammock'. The bladder neck is closed off as it is pulled backwards and downwards against an immobilized proximal urethra. This is achieved by stretching of the underlying vagina. Proper function of the pubo-urethral ligaments, vaginal hammock and pubo-coccygeus muscles are essential to achieve this.[6]

Intrinsic damage to the rhabdosphincter, or a scarred drainpipe urethra that cannot occlude properly, may occur after:

- vaginal surgery
- previous incontinence surgery
- urethral dilatation
- chronic urethritis
- radiotherapy.[7]

Electromyographic studies have demonstrated denervation of the intrinsic and extrinsic sphincter mechanisms.[8,9] Postmenopausal atrophy may affect the urethral sphincter.[10] The prevalence of all urinary incontinence (UI) increases with age. Such damage affects the hermetic closure properties of the proximal urethra, and USI may be the result.

> Electromyography has shown that both the intrinsic and extrinsic sphincter mechanisms are denervated in USI

Clinical features

Stress urinary incontinence (SUI) is the involuntary leakage of urine from the urethra. It is synchronous with effort or exertion, or sneezing or coughing.[2] The urine is usually lost in small amounts without any associated urgency. Twenty-five percent of incontinent women suffer incontinence during intercourse. Intercourse-related incontinence at penetration, rather than orgasm, is typical for women complaining of SUI.[11]

Overall, approximately one-half of all incontinent women complain of pure stress incontinence and 30–40% complain of mixed symptoms of stress and urge incontinence.[12]

> 50% of incontinent women complain of pure stress incontinence and 30–40% have mixed symptoms of urge and stress incontinence

Investigations

Frequency–volume chart

Frequency–volume charts give objective quantification of fluid intake, voiding frequency and functional bladder capacity.

Typical features of the frequency–volume chart of women with USI are a normal, or slightly increased, diurnal frequency without nocturia. Episodes of incontinence associated with physical activity or exertion, rather than urgency, are found.

Pad test

Pad tests are used to verify incontinence and to quantify the urine loss.[13] A pre-weighed perineal pad is placed into the individual's underwear. A series of standardized manoeuvres are then carried out, including coughing, climbing stairs and bending down. The patient then voids, and the volume is recorded. The pad is re-weighed – an increase greater than 1 g in one hour confirms incontinence, as anything less may be caused by discharge or sweat.

Urine culture

Urinary tract infection, especially in the elderly, will worsen bladder symptoms and invalidate urodynamic investigation. The presence of infection may mimic DO, and so lead to an inaccurate diagnosis and ineffective treatment.

> Infections of the urinary tract will make bladder symptoms worse and will invalidate urodynamic investigations

Urodynamics

Symptoms of lower urinary tract dysfunction are often misleading. 'Urodynamics' is a term used to describe a combination of tests of the ability of the bladder to store and expel urine.[14] Studies have repeatedly shown the greater value of urodynamics over symptoms alone in diagnostic accuracy.[15,16] Only 39% of women complaining of stress incontinence have USI.[17]

Video-urodynamics

Video-urodynamics combines fluoroscopic imaging of the bladder neck with cystometry by filling the bladder with iodine-based contrast medium. This allows differentiation between USI due to bladder-neck hypermobility and that due to intrinsic sphincter deficiency (ISD). In addition, anatomical variants can be identified.

Treatment

Conservative management

A conservative approach is often justified (Table 5.1), especially if symptoms are only mild or easily manageable. When a woman is planning on having more children, or when symptoms manifest during pregnancy, surgery should be avoided. Symptoms may be ameliorated by appropriate conservative interventions if:

● surgery is considered unwise because of medical illness

● surgery is refused

● the waiting time for surgery is long.

Physical therapies

The mainstay of treatment for USI in the UK is physiotherapy, with recourse to surgery when indicated and desired. Physiotherapy modalities include:

● pelvic-floor-muscle training

● electrical stimulation

● vaginal cones

● urethral devices

● use of biofeedback.

> Physiotherapy is the main form of treatment of USI in the UK – methods include electrical stimulation, vaginal cones, pelvic-floor-muscle training, biofeedback and urethral devices

Physical therapies represent the least invasive, but effective option for treating USI. For this reason they are commonly used as first-line

Table 5.1
Indications for conservative treatment of USI

● Mild or easily manageable symptoms
● Family incomplete
● Symptoms manifest during pregnancy
● Surgery contraindicated by coexisting medical conditions
● Surgery declined by patient
● Long waiting time for surgery

treatment. The advantage of this approach is that many women's symptoms are cured or improved to the point where they do not require surgery, with its potential complications. Additionally, the success rate of future operative procedures is not adversely affected – but this may occur following failed surgical treatment.

Pelvic floor exercises

Pelvic floor exercises (PFEs) provide, in addition to an increase in the strength and tone of the pelvic floor, enhancement of cortical awareness of muscle groups and hypertrophy of existing muscle fibres. Women need instruction, motivation and an understanding of the pelvic floor musculature before they begin PFEs.

> PFEs increase the strength and tone of the pelvic-floor muscles. They are more effective than no treatment and electrical stimulation at preventing incontinence

Teaching PFEs is one of the hardest things asked of the physiotherapist, as the muscles concerned are not visible. A large, simple diagram or model of the pelvis, pelvic organs and muscles is extremely useful. Language should be directed at the appropriate educational level.

The woman is asked to perform long, strong contractions of the pelvic floor, with a rest of about four seconds between each, to see how long each contraction can be held for, and how many repetitions can be achieved. The woman is also asked to perform short sharp repetitions until fatigued, and the result is recorded. The aim is to achieve an increase in the number and duration of contractions over the period of treatment.[18] Pelvic floor muscle training is more effective than no treatment, electrical stimulation and vaginal cones.[19]

In a study of 747 postnatal women randomized to either standard postnatal care or pelvic floor muscle training with regular assessment, fewer women in the study group had urinary incontinence at one year (59.9% vs 69%,

$p=0.037$). Severe incontinence was even further reduced (19.7% vs 31.8%, $p=0.002$).[20] However, at 5–7 years after delivery 44.6% of women admit to some urinary incontinence, with 4.1% having daily or more frequent leakage. There was a significant remission and new onset rate of urinary incontinence over the duration of the study, with just over 27% of the incontinent women in 1994 becoming dry in 2000, and 31.7% of the continent women in 1994 becoming incontinent in 2000.[21]

Vaginal cones

Resistance, in the form of weights, is used to increase muscle strength and endurance. This is true in the case of gym attendance and it applies equally to the pelvic floor. Vaginal cones were developed as a way of applying graded resistance against which the pelvic floor muscles may work. The theory of cone usage is of increased activity in the muscles to counteract gravity and downward movement.[18]

> Vaginal cones are thought to improve muscle activity to counteract gravity and downward movement

To overcome concerns regarding infection, cones are available for single-user use over the counter in the UK. At King's College Hospital we recommend that cones be used after instruction from a specialist physiotherapist.

A Cochrane review by Herbison et al[22] concluded that cones are better than no treatment, but that there were considerable drop-out rates in some studies.

Electrical stimulation

Electrical stimulation can be used for two purposes. It may assist in the production of muscle contractions in those women who either have an extremely weak contraction or are unable to produce a muscle contraction. It may also be used to inhibit DO by the sensory feedback it produces.[18] Many different devices have been used, including:

- vaginal
- perineal
- pudendal
- anal
- abdominal
- tibial
- implanted devices.

Those commonly used are the vaginal and rectal plug electrodes.

A study of home electrical stimulation, in combination with PFEs, showed an improvement over no treatment and PFE alone. There was no difference in outcome between the active arms of the study.[23]

Biofeedback

Biofeedback relies on the principle of relaying information about a normally subconscious physiological process to the conscious awareness of the individual. This information is relayed as an audible, tactile or visual signal and may be used to assist in modifying behaviour to control the signal appropriately.[24]

Drug therapy

Anecdotally, various agents such as α_1-adrenoreceptor agonists, oestrogens and tricyclic antidepressants have all been used for the management of urodynamic stress incontinence.

Recent drug trials

A new drug has been developed specifically for the treatment of stress incontinence. Duloxetine is the first and only drug licensed for the treatment of moderate to severe stress urinary incontinence. It is a relatively balanced serotonin (5-hydroxytryptamine) and noradrenaline reuptake inhibitor (SNRI) that enhances urethral striated sphincter activity via a centrally mediated pathway.[25] The efficacy and safety of duloxetine at various daily doses (20 mg, 40 mg, 80 mg) has been evaluated in several double-blind randomized studies.[26] Duloxetine was associated with significant and dose-dependent decreases in incontinence episode frequency. Reductions were 41% for placebo and 54%, 59% and 64% for the 20 mg, 40 mg, and 80 mg groups respectively. Discontinuation rates were also dose-dependent: 5% for placebo and 9%, 12% and 15% for 20 mg, 40 mg, and 80 mg respectively. The most frequently reported adverse event was nausea.

> Duloxetine, a new drug for stress incontinence, is an SNRI that enhances urethral striated sphincter activity via a centrally mediated pathway

A further global study of 458 women has also recently been reported.[27] There was a significant decrease in incontinence episode frequency and an improvement in quality-of-life in those women taking duloxetine 40 mg bd when compared with women taking placebo. Once again, nausea was the most frequently reported adverse event, occurring in 25.1% of women receiving duloxetine and 3.9% in those taking placebo. However, 60% of nausea resolved within seven days and 86% by one month.

These findings are supported by a further double-blind, placebo-controlled study of 109 women awaiting surgery for stress incontinence.[28] Overall, there was a significant improvement in incontinence episode frequency and quality-of-life in those women taking duloxetine when compared with placebo. Twenty percent of women who were awaiting continence surgery changed their mind whilst taking duloxetine.

> Studies of duloxetine have shown that it gives a significant improvement in incontinence episode frequency and quality-of-life compared with placebo

Recently introduced, duloxetine may be an effective addition to surgery and pelvic floor education in the management of women with moderate to severe stress incontinence. Indeed duloxetine in combination with pelvic floor education may be more effective than either treatment alone.

Surgery

When considering surgical treatment of urinary incontinence, it is important to be clear about the underlying cause as the effects of surgery are largely irreversible. Whereas USI is often successfully treated by surgical intervention, DO is not. Indeed, it may be made worse by incontinence surgery.

> USI can be successfully treated with surgery; however, DO cannot and is often made worse by surgery

The traditional aims of incontinence surgery were:

- to elevate the bladder neck and proximal urethra – to support them and prevent funnelling
- to align the bladder neck to the postero-superior aspect of the symphysis pubis – in order to increase outflow resistance.

In 1961 Burch published a paper describing a technique to support the urethra and bladder by elevation of the paravaginal tissue to the ipsilateral ileo-pectineal ligament.[29]

The Burch colposuspension has excellent long-term results[30] and is still regarded as the 'gold standard' against which new procedures are judged. Subjective success rates in excess of 90% have been reported. However, objective outcome measures, determined on the basis of postoperative urodynamic testing, are usually lower.[31]

> Burch colposuspension has excellent long-term results and is the 'gold standard' for incontinence surgery

Many surgical procedures have been described, with varying degrees of success. Comparison of 'cure' rates for these operations is often difficult for a number of reasons:

- The sensitivities of the different outcome

measures employed varied, and this influences the reported 'cure' rates.

- The type of population studied, appropriateness of patient selection and skill of the surgeon performing the procedure represent major confounding factors when comparing different studies.

Despite these difficulties, a series of useful meta-analyses have been published by Jarvis,[31] Black and Downs,[32] and the American Urological Association.[33] These allow comparisons to be made between different operations (Table 5.2); it has resulted in a number of procedures that were previously widely used for the surgical treatment of USI (such as the anterior repair and needle suspensions) being abandoned because of poor objective long-term results.[34]

Sling procedures

Suburethral sling procedures were initially developed in the 1880s. Overall, sling procedures, using autologous or synthetic materials, produce a continence rate of approximately 80% and an improvement rate of 90%, with little reduction in continence over time. They are associated with a high incidence of voiding difficulties and detrusor overactivity.[35] Synthetic sling materials are also associated with erosion into the vagina or urinary tract.[36]

> Sling procedures produce a continence rate of 80% and an improvement rate of 90%, with little reduction in continence over time

Morbidity

One must consider the risks of morbidity and mortality when counselling regarding surgery, and be aware of the risks of *de novo* DO and voiding difficulty,[37] failure of the procedure, and future recurrence. Over the past 20 years, attention has been directed at developing less invasive procedures, which replicate the high cure rates of slings and the Burch colposuspension[32] but with reduced morbidity, reduced hospital stay and shorter time taken to return to normal activities. Three types of surgical intervention characterize the current trend towards less invasive surgical treatments for female stress urinary incontinence:

- laparoscopic colposuspension
- mid-urethral tape procedures
  - tension-free vaginal tape (TVT)
  - SPARC female sling system
  - transobturator tapes (TOT)
  - intravaginal slingplasty (IVS)
- injectable peri-urethral bulking agents.

Laparoscopic colposuspension

This technique was first described by Vancaillie in 1991. Theoretically, if the operation is the same as an open Burch procedure, the same long-term success rates should be obtained but with reduced morbidity and quicker recovery.[38]

Six randomized controlled trials have been published comparing the laparoscopic and open approaches to colposuspension. A diverse range of techniques has been described, with a correspondingly wide variety of reported cure rates.

Table 5.2
Objective cure rates for first procedure and recurrent incontinence[31]

Procedure	First procedure		Recurrent incontinence	
	Mean (%)	95% CI	Mean (%)	95% CI
Slings	93.9	89.2–98.6	86.1	82.4–89.8
Burch colposuspension	89.8	87.6–92.1	82.5	76.3–88.7
Needle suspension	86.7	75.5–97.9	86.4	72.4–100
Anterior vaginal repair	67.8	62.9–72.8	N/A	N/A
Injectables	45.5	28.5–62.5	57.8	43.2–72.4

It does seem clear that there is a considerable 'learning curve' associated with laparoscopic colposuspension.[39] At five years, the rate of demonstrable USI on videocystourethography was only 10% in the open group, compared with 43% in the laparoscopic group. In contrast, those studies in which an experienced endoscopic surgeon performed the procedure report no significant difference in outcome.[40] It has been suggested that optimal results cannot be achieved until experience of around 50 cases has accrued.

There is no logical reason why, if they are performed identically, the success rate of laparoscopic Burch should be different from the open procedure. The important factors appear to be the laparoscopic experience of the surgeon and the type of suture used. Currently, the long-term performance of laparoscopic colposuspension is uncertain. Despite a quicker recovery, the operation takes longer to perform, is associated with more surgical complications and is more expensive.[41]

> Although there is a quicker recovery time with laparoscopic colposuspension, it is a longer operation with more surgical complication and is more expensive than Burch colposuspension

The tension-free vaginal tape procedure

The development of the tension-free vaginal tape (TVT) procedure was based on experimental and clinical studies undertaken by Petros and Ulmsten. They described the anatomy and function of the female pelvic floor and the urethral closure mechanism. The central theme of the theory is that the vagina acts as a 'hammock' with two distinct anatomical segments. These segments are pulled in opposite directions against the pubo-urethral ligament, which acts as a fulcrum. The bladder neck is closed off as it is pulled backwards and downwards against an immobilized proximal urethra. This is achieved by stretching of the underlying vagina. Proper function of the pubo-urethral ligaments, vaginal hammock and pubo-coccygeus muscles are essential to achieve this.[42] Operating on almost 100 women over a 12-month period, Petros and Ulmsten achieved an 84% subjective and objective cure rate at two years with no long-term voiding difficulties or de novo DO.[43] This concept has since been developed into the TVT (Gynecare).

TVT has some similarity to conventional sling techniques. However, the TVT is placed under the mid-urethra via a small vaginal incision, using local, regional or general anaesthesia. Postoperative discomfort is minimal and most women can return to normal activity within two weeks.

> TVT is placed under the mid-urethra via a small vaginal incision. Postoperative discomfort is minimal

To date the longest follow-up studies available are those from Scandinavia, where the procedure was first performed. There are several publications showing continued efficacy of TVT up to five years postoperatively. Nilsson et al reported a subjective and objective cure rate of 85% in a series of 90 patients, 85 of whom were followed up to a median of 56 months.[44]

A recent randomized, multicentre study carried out in the UK compared the TVT with the Burch colposuspension.[45,46] The study was undertaken in 14 centres and recruited 344 women. The primary outcome measures used were negative cystometry and perineal pad testing at six months and pad testing alone at 12 and 24 months. In addition, clinical, urodynamic, quality-of-life and health economic secondary outcome measures were studied. The data were analysed on the basis that missing data were treated as failures. At six months the results were similar in each treatment group, with objective cure rates of 68% for TVT and 66% for colposuspension. Interestingly, while the efficacy of both procedures remained compatible across a range of different subjective and objective outcome measures, the trial highlighted considerable variation in cure rates depending upon which outcome measure is used to define 'cure'. At two years follow-up the cure rates remained similar in each treatment arm. Sixty-five percent of the TVT group and 59% of the colposuspension group were found to be dry on pad testing. There were no statistically significant differences in any of the outcome parameters up to two years.

Injectable periurethral bulking agents

Injectable agents have a lower immediate success rate than other procedures, and in the long term there is a continued decline in continence. Most reports quote 60–80% initial improvement rates, but this falls to around 40% of women remaining dry after two years.[47] However, the procedure has a low morbidity and may have a role after other procedures have failed.

> Injectable periurethral bulking agents have a lower immediate success rate than other methods and there is also a long-term continued decline in continence. However, the procedure does have a low morbidity

The most commonly used periurethral bulking agents in current use are:

- glutaraldehyde cross-linked bovine collagen (Contigen, Bard Ltd)
- macroparticulate silicone particles (Macroplastique, Uroplasty Ltd).

Glutaraldehyde bovine collagen

Glutaraldehyde cross-linked bovine collagen has not been shown to have any side-effects due to migration. However, due to the significant reabsorption of this material over time, repeated injections may be necessary to sustain continence.

Silicone particles

The other commonly used injectable consists of micronized silicone rubber particles suspended

in a non-silicone carrier gel. The larger particle size of this material makes migration and displacement less likely. The silicone particles are designed to act as a bulking agent, with local inflammatory response removing the carrier gel. This results in encapsulation of the silicon in fibrin and replacement of the gel with collagen fibres. Reported cure rates with Macroplastique are similar to those with Contigen, but less of the material is required. Agents may be injected either transurethrally via a cystoscope or paraurethrally under cystoscopic control. Recently, devices that allow injections to be made without the use of a cystoscope have been introduced. These enable periurethral injections to be given under local anaesthetic, in an outpatient clinic.

> The two main injectable agents used are glutaraldehyde cross-linked bovine collagen and micronized silicone rubber particles that are suspended in a non-silicone carrier gel

Trials

Studies using these agents report 'cure' rates in the region of 40–60%,[48,49] with re-injection rates as high as 22% within two years after attaining initial dryness.[50]

Although the low complication rate of injectable bulking agents makes their use appear attractive, it is their poor long-term success that limits their use. Few well-conducted, long-term studies have been published. Given such poor long-term results, the use of this technique as a first-line treatment in fit, younger women is difficult to justify. Injectables are invaluable, however, in:

- the frail elderly
- the treatment of secondary incontinence in women who have undergone multiple failed procedures
- cases where the urethra is fixed and scarred after radiotherapy.

Summary

A brief examination of the history of incontinence surgery reveals that a wide variety of different techniques have been developed, which were initially enthusiastically adopted, only for it to be found that longer-term results were often disappointing. It is only comparatively recently that reliable data have been available on efficacy and complication rates for many of these procedures. It is therefore important that all new surgical procedures undergo comprehensive evaluation, including accurate reporting of complications, prior to being adopted for widespread use. This is best achieved by large-scale randomized trials, with long-term follow-up, comparing new procedures with tried and tested surgical treatments.

Many of the newer surgical procedures for treating urinary incontinence appear to offer improved safety and shorter hospital admissions than traditional open incontinence surgery. This should not undermine the fundamental importance of appropriate preoperative investigation. The increasing range of available procedures allows treatment to be individualized. Definitive surgery is most appropriate for younger active women, whereas those techniques offering reduced morbidity, possibly at the cost of poorer long-term efficacy, may be more appropriate in some older women. Thorough assessment and careful counselling should allow all women a choice of safe, effective treatment for USI.

References

1. Hunskaar S, Lose G, Sykes D, Voss S. The prevalence of urinary incontinence in women in four European countries. *BJU International* 2004; **93**: 324–30.

2. Abrams P, Cardozo L, Fall M *et al.* The standardisation of terminology of lower urinary tract function: report from the Standardisation Sub-Committee of the International Continence Society. *Neurourol Urodyn* 2002; **21**: 167–78.

3. Enhorning GE. A concept of urinary continence. *Urol Int* 1976; **31**: 3–5.

4. Greenwald SW, Thorbury JR, Dunn LJ. Cystourethrography as an aid in stress incontinence. *Obstet Gynecol* 1967; **29**: 324.

5. Constantinou CE, Govan DE. Contribution and timing of transmitted and generated pressure components in the female urethra. *Prog Clin Biol Res* 1981; **78**: 113–20.

6. Petros PE, Ulmsten UI. An integral theory of female urinary incontinence. Experimental and clinical considerations. *Acta Obstet Gynecol Scand Suppl* 1990; **153**: 7–31.

7. Keller C. Epidemiology and classification of incontinence. In: Cardozo LD (ed). *Urogynaecology*. Edinburgh: Churchill Livingstone, 1997, pp 3–23.

8. Smith AR, Hosker GL, Warrell DW. The role of pudendal nerve damage in the aetiology of genuine stress incontinence in women. *Br J Obstet Gynaecol* 1989; **96**: 29–32.

9. Allen RE, Hosker GL, Smith AR, Warrell DW. Pelvic floor damage and childbirth: a neurophysiological study. *Br J Obstet Gynaecol* 1990; **97**: 770–9.

10. Fantl JA, Cardozo L, McClish DK. Estrogen therapy in the management of urinary incontinence in post-menopausal women: a meta-analysis. First report of the Hormones and Urogenital Therapy Committee. *Obstet Gynecol* 1994; **83**: 12–18.

11. Hilton P. Urinary incontinence during sexual intercourse: a common, but rarely volunteered, symptom. *Br J Obstet Gynaecol* 1988; **95**: 377–81.

12. Hannestad YS, Rortveit G, Sandvik H, Hunskaar S. A community-based epidemiological survey of female urinary incontinence: the Norwegian EPINCONT study. Epidemiology of incontinence in the County of Nord-Trondelag. *J Clin Epidemiol* 2000; **53**: 1150–7.

13. Sutherst JL, Brown M, Shawer M. Assessing the severity of urge incontinence in women by weighing perineal pads. *Lancet* 1981; **i**: 1128–30.

14. Hosker G. ICS (UK) Annual Scientific Meeting, Leicester. April 2003. Expert presentation.

15. Jarvis GJ, Hall S, Stamp S, Millar DR. An assessment of urodynamic investigation in incontinent women. *Br J Obstet Gynaecol* 1980; **87**: 873–96.

16. James M, Jackson S, Shepherd A, Abrams P. Pure stress leakage symptomatology: is it safe to discount detrusor instability? *Br J Obstet Gynaecol* 1999; **106**: 1255–8.

17. Abrams P. The clinical contribution of urodynamics. In: Abrams P, Feneley R, Torrens M (eds). *Urodynamics*. Berlin: Springer-Verlag, 1983, pp 118–74.

18. Mantle J. Urinary Function and Dysfunction. In: Mantle J, Haslam J, Barton S. *Physiotherapy in Obstetrics and Gynaecology, 2nd Edition*. Oxford: Butterworth Heinemann, 2004, pp 333–82.

19. Bo K, Talseth T, Holme I. Single blind, randomised controlled trial of pelvic floor exercises, electrical stimulation, vaginal cones, and no treatment in management of genuine stress incontinence in women. *Br Med J* 1999; **318**: 487–93.

20. Glazener CM, Herbison GP, Wilson PD *et al.* Conservative management of persistent postnatal urinary and faecal incontinence: randomised controlled trial. *Br Med J* 2001; **323**: 593–6.

21. Wilson PD, Herbison P, Glazener C et al. Obstetric practice and urinary incontinence 5-7 years after delivery. *Neurourol Urodynam* 2002; **21**: 284–300.

22. Herbison P, Plevnik S, Mantle J. Weighted vaginal cones for urinary incontinence. In: The Cochrane Library, Issue 1. Update Software, Oxford.

23. Parsons M, Mantle J, Cardozo L et al. A single blind, randomised, controlled trial of pelvic floor muscle training with home electrical stimulation in the treatment of urodynamic stress incontinence. Unpublished data.

24. Cardozo LD, Abrams P, Stanton SL, Fennelly RCL. Idiopathic detrusor instability treated by biofeedback. *Br J Urol* 1978; **50**: 24–9.

25. Thor KB, Katofiasc MA. Effects of duloxetine, a combined serotonin and norepinephrine reuptake inhibitor, on central neural control of lower urinary tract function in the chloralose-anesthetised female cat. *J Pharmacol Exp Ther* 1995; **274**: 1014–24.

26. Norton PA, Zinner NR, Yalcin I, Bump RC. Duloxetine Urinary Incontinence Study Group. Duloxetine versus placebo in the treatment of stress urinary incontinence. *Am J Obstet Gynaecol* 2002; **187**: 40–8.

27. Millard R, Moore K, Yalcin I, Bump R. Duloxetine vs. placebo in the treatment of stress urinary incontinence: a global phase III study. *Nerourol Urodynam* 2003; **22**: 482–3.

28. Drutz H, Cardozo L, Baygani S, Bump R. Duloxetine treatment of women with only urodynamic stress incontinence awaiting continence surgery. *Neurourol Urodynam* 2003; **22**: 523–4.

29. Burch JC. Urethrovesical fixation to Cooper's ligament for correction of stress incontinence, cystocele and prolapse. *Am J Obstet Gynaecol* 1961; **81**: 281–90.

30. Alcalay M, Monga A, Stanton SL. Burch colposuspension: a 10–20 year follow up. *Br J Obstet Gynaecol* 1995; **102**: 740–5.

31. Jarvis GJ. Surgery for stress incontinence. *Br J Obstet Gynaecol* 1994; **101**: 371–4.

32. Black NA, Downs SH. The effectiveness of surgery for stress incontinence in women: a systematic review. *Br J Urol* 1996; **78**: 497–510.

33. Leach G, Dmochowski R, Appell R et al. Female stress urinary incontinence guidlines. Panel summary report on surgical management of female stress urinary incontinence. *J Urol* 1997; **158**: 875–80.

34. Kevelighan EH, Aagaard J, Balasubramaniam B, Jarvis GJ. The Stamey endoscopic bladder neck suspension – a 10 year follow-up study. *Br J Obstet Gynaecol* 1998; **105 (Suppl 17)**: 47.

35. Bidmead J, Cardozo L. Sling techniques in the treatment of genuine stress incontinence. *Br J Obstet Gynaecol* 2000; **107**: 147–56.

36. Jarvis GJ. Stress incontinence. In: Mundy AR,Stephenson TP,Wein AJ (eds). *Urodynamics*. Edinburgh: Churchill Livingstone, 1994, pp 299–326.

37. Bombieri L, Freeman RM, Perkins EP et al. Why do women have voiding dysfunction and de novo detrusor instability after colposuspension? *Br J Obstet Gynaecol* 2002; **109**: 402–12.

38. Vancaillie TG, Schuessler W. Laparoscopic bladderneck suspension. *J Laparoendosc Surg* 1991; **1**: 169–73.

39. Burton G. A five year prospective randomised urodynamic study comparing open and laparoscopic colposuspension. *Neurol Urodyn* 1999; **18**: 295–6.

40. Morris A, Reilly E, Hassan A et al. 5–7 year follow up of a randomised trial comparing laparoscopic colposuspension and open colposuspension in the treatment of genuine stress incontinence. *Int Urogynecol J* 2001; **12**: S6–S7.

41. Moehrer B, Ellis G, Carey M, Wilson PD. Laparoscopic colposuspension for urinary incontinence in women. *Cochrane Database Syst Rev* 2002; **1**: CD002239.

42. Petros PE, Ulmsten UI. An integral theory of female urinary incontinence. Experimental and clinical considerations. *Acta Obstet Gynecol Scand Suppl* 1990; **153**: 7–31.

43. Ulmsten U, Henriksson L, Johnson P, Varhos G. An ambulatory surgical procedure under local anaesthesia for treatment of female urinary incontinence. *Int Urogynecol J* 1996; **7**: 81–6.

44. Nilsson C, Kuuva N, Falconer C et al. Long-term of the tension-free vaginal tape (TVT) procedure for surgical treatment of female stress urinary incontinence. *Int Urogynecol J Pelvic Floor Dysfunct* 2001; **12(Suppl 2)**: S5–S8.

45. Ward K, Hilton P, Browning J. A randomised trial of colposuspension and tension free vaginal tape (TVT) for primary genuine stress incontinence. *Neurourol Urodyn* 2000; **19**: 386–7.

46. Ward KL, Hilton P: A randomised trial of colposuspension and tension-free vaginal tape (TVT) for primary genuine stress incontinence–2 year follow-up. *Int Urogynecol J Pelvic Floor Dysfunct* 2001; **12(Suppl 1)**: S7–8.

47. Monga AK, Robinson D, Stanton SL. Peri-urethral collagen injections for genuine stress incontinence: a two-year follow-up. *Br J Urol* 1995; **76**: 156–60.

48. Khullar V, Cardozo LD, Abbott D, Anders K. GAX collagen in the treatment of urinary incontinence in elderly women: a two year follow-up. *Br J Obstet Gynaecol* 1997; **104**: 96–9.

49. Radley SC, Chapple CR, Mitsogiannis IC, Glass KS. Transurethral implantation of macroplastique for the treatment of female stress urinary incontinence secondary to urethral sphincter deficiency. *Eur Urol* 2001; **39**: 383–9.

50. Winters JC, Appell RA. Injection of collagen in the treatment of intrinsic sphincter deficiency in the female patient. *Urol Clin North Am* 1995; **22**: 673–8.

6. Detrusor overactivity

Introduction
Definition
Pathophysiology and aetiology
Clinical features
Investigation
Non-drug treatment
Drug therapy
Surgical management
Summary

Introduction

Detrusor overactivity (DO) is the second commonest cause of urinary incontinence (UI). It occurs in 20–40% of those women referred for urodynamic investigation and may be present in up to 10% of the general population. The incidence of DO increases with age, and urge incontinence is the most common symptom of incontinence in those over 60 years[1] and in the elderly.[2] Urodynamic assessment is required to make an accurate diagnosis of DO, as women usually present with multiple symptoms, the most common of which is urgency with or without frequency and/or incontinence.

> Urodynamic assessment is essential when making a diagnosis of DO as women often present with multiple symptoms

Definition

Detrusor overactivity is a urodynamic observation characterized by involuntary detrusor contractions during the filling phase. The contractions may be spontaneous or provoked,[3] while the subject is actively trying to inhibit micturition. There is no lower limit for the amplitude of the contractions – rather they must be associated with symptoms of urge or desire to void. Interpretation of low-amplitude pressure changes depends on high-quality urodynamic technique.

Pathophysiology and aetiology

There are two main theories regarding the aetiology and pathophysiology of DO. It is thought to be either:

- a distortion or disruption of central control of the bladder
- a peripheral abnormality.

Centrally the problem may be one of reduced or absent inhibition of the voiding reflex caused by excessive suprapontine excitation, or reduced suprapontine inhibition. Peripherally, there may be excessive cholinergic excitation or reduced neuropeptidergic inhibition.

> DO may be caused by either a peripheral abnormality or a distortion or disruption of central control of the bladder

Reasons for proposing a central causation for DO are that bladder control is a learnt phenomenon, which some individuals seem never to acquire. There is an association between mental anxiety and urinary frequency, seen in normal subjects under stressful conditions. There is a significant improvement in symptoms of DO when bladder retraining programmes are undertaken.[4,5]

Others believe that DO is caused by an abnormality of the detrusor muscle itself. Detrusor muscle from affected individuals shows an increased response to direct electrical stimulation and to stimulation with acetylcholine, compared with normal controls.[6]

Secondary causes

DO in men is often secondary to bladder outflow obstruction caused by prostatic hypertrophy. This is thought to result in a reduction in the number of smooth muscle fibres and an increase in the collagen content of the bladder.[7] However, as bladder outflow obstruction is uncommon in women, this is unlikely to play a significant role in the aetiology of idiopathic DO in females.

> Bladder outflow obstruction is uncommon in women so is unlikely to be a cause of idiopathic DO in females

A small number of cases occur secondary to pelvic surgery, often after surgery for stress incontinence.[8] This may be due to:

- trauma at the time of surgery
- the partially obstructive nature of most continence procedures.

DO is frequently found in the presence of neurological disease, such as multiple sclerosis, spina bifida or upper motor neurone lesions caused by trauma to the spinal cord. In these cases, it is known as neurogenic DO and can be particularly severe. Bladder problems are often the presenting feature in women with multiple sclerosis.

> Women with neurological diseases frequently have DO. Such diseases include spina bifida, multiple sclerosis or upper motor neurone lesions

Unknown aetiology

The aetiology of most cases of DO is unknown. Such 'idiopathic' DO may be secondary to poorly learned toilet training as an infant, especially in those who complain of lifelong symptoms. Alternatively, maladaptive behaviour may be learnt as an adult or may be secondary to psychological disturbance. Detrusor overactivity may also coexist with stress incontinence due to urethral sphincter incompetence. In these cases, the incontinence is termed 'mixed'. Symptoms of either condition may predominate and it may be difficult to determine the major pathology.

Clinical features

Revised definitions have recently been published by the International Continence Society:

- Lower urinary tract symptoms 'are the subjective indicator of a disease or change in condition as perceived by the patient, carer or partner and may lead him/her to seek help from the healthcare professional'.[3]
- Increased daytime frequency is the complaint by the patient who considers that he/she voids too often by day (equivalent to pollakisuria, which is used in many countries).
- Nocturia is the complaint that the individual has to wake at night one or more times to void.
- Urgency is the complaint of a sudden compelling desire (that is difficult to defer) to pass urine.
- Urge urinary incontinence is the complaint of involuntary leakage accompanied by, or immediately preceded by, a strong desire to void. Urgency, with or without urge incontinence, usually with frequency and nocturia, can be described as the overactive bladder syndrome, urge syndrome, or urgency–frequency syndrome.

> The ICS has recently published revised definitions of the clinical features of DO; see reference 3

Major symptoms

The prime symptoms of DO are urinary urgency, frequency of micturition and urge incontinence. Women who have a lack of bladder sensation may complain of urinary leakage without warning. Detrusor contractions may be provoked by rises in intraabdominal pressure – these can be caused by coughing, leading to a complaint of stress incontinence. Coital or orgasmic incontinence is also a feature of DO.[9]

> Coital or orgasmic incontinence is a feature of detrusor overactivity

There is considerable overlap of symptoms between women with DO and those with urodynamic stress incontinence (USI)[10] such that symptomatology may not be relied upon to accurately diagnose either condition. In one study[11] urgency and urge incontinence were found to have a sensitivity of 77.9% but a specificity of only 38.7% for DO. Approximately 34.9% of women complaining solely of USI were found to have DO. The likelihood of women having DO increases as the number of appropriate symptoms increases, with 89% probability of DO being diagnosed in the presence of all four major symptoms.[12]

Investigation

Medical and behavioural therapies for DO are often expensive and time-consuming. Accurate diagnosis helps aid uptake and compliance by ensuring that the right people are offered the right treatments. Full details of the assessment of incontinence are to be found in Chapter 3.

Frequency–volume chart

Frequency–volume charts give objective quantification of fluid intake, voiding frequency and functional bladder capacity. Urinary incontinence and episodes of urgency should also be documented. Typical features of DO are an increased diurnal urinary frequency associated with urgency and episodes of urge incontinence. Nocturia is one of the most salient features of DO.

Pad test

Pad testing may be appropriate to quantify the urinary loss. This test will not assess or document other symptoms of DO, such as urgency, which have a detrimental affect on quality-of-life.

> Although pad testing can quantify urine loss, it is not useful for assessing the other symptoms of DO

Urine culture

The symptoms of DO overlap with those of urinary tract infection (UTI). The presence of UTI will worsen irritative bladder symptoms and invalidate the results of urodynamic investigations. Exclusion of infection is therefore mandatory.

Urodynamics

Urodynamic studies are a measurement of the bladder's ability to store and expel urine[13] and are performed to differentiate between the various causes of incontinence. The diagnosis of DO can only be made after performing cystometry.

Video-urodynamics

A significant rise in intravesical pressure may lead to vesico-ureteric reflux and subsequent renal damage. This is especially common in women with neurogenic bladder problems. It is therefore important to be aware of any abnormalities in the renal tract, and the presence of vesico-ureteric reflux. This may be visualized by radiological screening during cystometry in either the filling or voiding phase.

Ambulatory urodynamics

This test is thought to be more physiological as non-provocative filling is used, and during the period of the test the woman may go about 'normal' activities (eg walking, using stairs) – perhaps including those that cause her to be incontinent. It is thought to be a more sensitive test than laboratory urodynamics, detecting an extra 30% of cases of DO. The recordings of ambulatory urodynamics are analysed in the same way, with attention being directed at the correlation between pressure recordings and symptoms.

> Ambulatory urodynamics is more sensitive than laboratory urodynamics, and detects an extra 30% of DO cases

Non-drug treatment

Not all women will require treatment for their DO. For some, simple reassurance and lifestyle interventions with behavioural modification may suffice. For others, it is appropriate to undertake initial investigation, with advice on simple lifestyle changes and perhaps empirical treatment, prior to referral to secondary care (Table 6.1).

Behavioural therapy

Caffeine has been shown to increase the 'irritability' of the bladder in those who have DO.[14] It is therefore wise to moderate tea, coffee and cola intake, as well as alcohol – especially white wine. Limitation of fluid intake to 1–1.5 litres per day will also lessen the severity of symptoms. Various drugs, such as diuretics and antipsychotics, affect bladder function and their use should be reviewed.

> Caffeine 'irritates' the bladder; therefore, women with DO should moderate their tea, coffee and cola intake

For those requiring more than these simple measures, a variety of treatments exists. It is usually wise to start with the simplest of conservative therapies and progress through to treatments that are more radical if necessary.

Conservative management includes bladder retraining and other behavioural therapies.

Table 6.1
Conservative measures

- Fluid restriction (1.0–1.5 litres per day)
- Treat/exclude urinary tract infection
- Alter medication
- Behavioural interventions
  - bladder drill
  - biofeedback
  - hypnotherapy
- Treat chronic conditions, such as cough or constipation
- Timed/double voiding
- Weight reduction
- Catheters/pads/pants

Surgery is generally only used in women for whom these approaches have failed. Objective urodynamic assessment of the lower urinary tract, to establish a firm diagnosis, is mandatory prior to any incontinence surgery being performed. It is also used when simple measures have failed to offer adequate relief from symptoms, and further complex treatment is being contemplated.

Conservative therapy

Bladder retraining

Bladder control is usually learned as an infant during 'potty training'. The rationale behind bladder retraining is that maladaptive behaviour has been subsequently acquired in later life, and that if the bladder can be re-educated, continence can be restored. Several approaches to bladder retraining exist, including:

- bladder drill
- biofeedback
- maximal electrical stimulation (MES)
- hypnotherapy.

Bladder drill has been used for many years as a tool for treating urge incontinence[15] in the belief that DO is exacerbated, or even caused, by underlying psychological problems. Many women with DO link its onset to a particular life event.[16] The regimen used is usually that described by Jarvis and Millar:[17]

- exclude pathology and admit to hospital (if possible)
- explain the rationale to the patient
- instruct to void every 1.5 hours during the day; she must not void in between these times – either she waits or is incontinent
- when 1.5 hours is achieved, increase by half an hour and continue with 2-hourly voids
- normal fluid intake
- fluid chart kept by the patient
- encouragement from medical and nursing staff.

> After bladder drill, 90% of women with idiopathic DO become continent and 83% of these women will remain continent at six moths

Up to 90% of women with idiopathic DO may become continent with inpatient bladder drill, with 83% of these remaining continent after six months.[17] It is useful in the treatment of older women with all diagnoses,[18] and may avoid the need for drug treatment. Subjective improvement usually precedes cystometric improvement by up to three months. Women without DO on the cystometrogram are no less likely to relapse than those with cystometrically proven overactivity. Repeating bladder drill after relapse is less likely to be helpful, and some individuals may find other treatment modalities more useful.

Biofeedback

Biofeedback relies on the principle of relaying information about a normally subconscious physiological process to the conscious awareness of the individual. This information is relayed as an audible, tactile or visual signal. It can be used to assist in modifying behaviour to control the signal appropriately.[19] Initial cure/improvement rates of 80% have been quoted, but the relapse rate is high.[20] The treatment is time-intensive and requires a great deal of motivation from both the woman and the medical/nursing staff.

Maximal electrical stimulation

Maximal electrical stimulation (MES) involves stimulation of the pelvic floor muscles using electrodes. Many different devices have been used, including:

- vaginal
- perineal
- pudendal
- anal
- abdominal
- tibial
- implanted devices.

Those commonly used are the vaginal and rectal plug electrodes. Stimulation of afferent sensory pudendal fibres leads to inhibition of efferent motor impulses to the bladder, resulting in abolition of spontaneous detrusor contractions. Maximal response from MES is obtained by alternating pulses and intermittent stimulation so that muscle fatigue does not occur. The patient is taught to increase the stimulus strength to just below the level of discomfort. Objective success rates of 77% have been reported after one year.[21]

> Maximal electrical stimulation involves stimulation of the pelvic floor muscles using vaginal and rectal plug electrodes. This method aims to abolish spontaneous detrusor contractions

Hypnotherapy

Hypnotherapy has been reported as being successful in the treatment of some cases of DO.[22] Unfortunately, the relapse rate is very high. Few controlled trials have been performed, and there may be a large element of placebo response. It is not available on the NHS.

Acupuncture

Acupuncture is thought to work by raising levels of enkephalins and endorphins in the cerebrospinal fluid. Initial results have shown marked symptomatic improvement; however, this is not borne out by cystometric changes, and the benefits, as with many other behavioural therapies, seem to be short-lived.[23]

Summary

In summary, good initial results are often obtained from behavioural therapies, but they require a high level of motivation from both the patient and the medical/nursing staff. Improvement is often not maintained, and a large placebo response element is probably involved.

Drug therapy

Most women with DO will require drug therapy. Many drugs have been tried in the treatment of DO – none is completely satisfactory, and many have had to be abandoned due to lack of efficacy, or dangerous or unpleasant side-effects. For many of the drugs, their clinical use is based on weak, open studies rather than randomized controlled trials. (Table 6.2 shows the levels of evidence of efficacy available for some drugs.) Even then, the placebo response is so large that clinical effect is difficult to distinguish.[24]

> Many incontinence drugs have been abandoned due to lack of efficacy and dangerous/unpleasant side-effects

Drug effects in individuals, however, can vary markedly. Even those drugs presently in use are not without their problems. Most of these drugs exert their effect by acting on the acetylcholine receptors within the detrusor muscle; other drugs have central effects, act to reduce urine production or raise the sensory threshold of the bladder. As they are not without side-effects, therapy is seldom continued indefinitely, and so must be considered as an adjunct to behavioural therapy.

> Drug therapy should be considered an adjct to behavioural therapy due to the side-effects caused by the medication

The use of drugs in the frail, elderly and infirm is contentious. Much lower doses of drugs should be used in the frail and elderly. Alcohol and medication use are major causes of acute incontinence in the elderly. Polypharmacy and the use of psychotropic medication are most prevalent in women aged 85 years or over, and the number appears to be increasing,[25] thereby compounding the problem.

Antimuscarinic (anticholinergic) agents

The main transmitter in the parasympathetic nervous system is acetylcholine. Voluntary and

Table 6.2
Drugs used in the treatment of DO[34]. Levels of evidence and assessment with recommendations (see Appendix B)

	Level of evidence	Grade of recommendation
Antimuscarinic drugs		
Tolterodine	1	A
Trospium	1	A
Propantheline	2	B
Atropine, hyoscyamine	2	D
Darifenacin, solifenacin	Under investigation	
Drugs acting on membrane channels		
Calcium-channel antagonists	Under investigation	
Potassium-channel openers	Under investigation	
Drugs with mixed actions		
Oxybutynin	1	A
Propiverine	1	A
Dicyclomine	4	C
Flavoxate	4	D
Alpha-blockers		
Alfuzosin	4	D
Doxazosin	4	D
Prazosin	4	D
Terazosin	4	D
Tamsulosin	4	D
Beta-agonists		
Terbutaline	4	D
Clenbuterol	4	D
Salbutamol	4	D
Antidepressants		
Imipramine	2	C (with caution)
Amitriptylline	3	
Prostaglandin synthesis inhibitors		
Indomethacin	4	C
Flurbiprofen	4	C
Vasopressin analogues		
Desmopressin	1	A
Other drugs		
Baclofen	2*	C*
Capsaicin	3	C
Resiniferatoxin	Under investigation	

*Intrathecal use

involuntary bladder contractions are mediated via muscarinic receptors in the bladder smooth muscle. Antimuscarinic agents act by competitive inhibition at the postganglionic receptor sites and therefore suppress both types of contraction, irrespective of the activation of the efferent part of the reflex.

Atropine and other related compounds are tertiary amines. Unfortunately, they are easily absorbed from the gastrointestinal (GI) tract and pass readily into the central nervous system (CNS) so CNS side-effects, such as drowsiness are common. The side-effects caused by atropine can be so severe that they prevent its use in clinical practice; but other drugs, such as propantheline, have been quite commonly used.

> Atropine and other tertiary amines commonly cause CNS side-effects

Quaternary amines, on the other hand, are not readily absorbed from the GI tract, and do not readily pass into the CNS. Therefore they have have fewer central side-effects. They still produce marked peripheral antimuscarinic effects:

- accommodation paralysis
- blurred vision
- dry mouth
- tachycardia
- constipation.

All antimuscarinics are contraindicated in acute (narrow angle) glaucoma.

Tolterodine

Tolterodine is a potent and competitive muscarinic receptor antagonist. It has no selectivity for the subtypes of muscarinic receptor, but seems to show selectivity for the bladder over the salivary glands.[26] The therapeutic effect of tolterodine is bolstered by the similar activity of the metabolite.[27,28] Although tolterodine is rapidly absorbed and has a half-life of only 2–3 hours, the clinical benefits in the bladder may last rather longer, due to the presence of pharmacologically active metabolites.[28] In healthy volunteers, suppression of salivation

was much shorter than inhibition of micturition after high-dose administration.[26] Tolterodine does not readily cross the blood–brain barrier, and so has a low incidence of cognitive side-effects.

> Tolterodine has a low incidence of cognitive side-effects as it does not readily cross the blood–brain barrier

The most frequently cited troublesome side-effect is dry mouth, occurring in 28% of individuals in one study.[29] In this study only 70% were able to continue treatment for nine months and 9% withdrew due to adverse events.

An extended-release formulation of tolterodine (tolterodine ER) has been developed. In a large, double-blind, multicentre, randomized study, a once-daily preparation of tolterodine ER 4 mg was compared with immediate-release tolterodine 2 mg bd and placebo. Both preparations were significantly better than placebo in treating the symptoms of DO. However, tolterodine ER was 18% more effective than the immediate-release preparation, with a 23% lower rate of dry mouth.[30] Tolterodine and oxybutynin immediate-release preparations have equal benefit in reducing incontinence episodes and urinary frequency,[31] but the side-effect profile favours tolterodine.

> The extended-release preparation of tolteridone appears to be more effective than the immediate-release version; it also has a lower rate of dry mouth, which is a common side-effect

Trospium

Trospium chloride is a quaternary ammonium compound, with antimuscarinic effects on smooth muscle. It has no selectivity for muscarinic receptor subtypes and has a low bioavailability. However, in studies on isolated detrusor muscle it was more potent than oxybutynin and tolterodine in blocking carbachol-induced contractions.[32] In a double-blind, controlled, multicentre study comparing trospium and oxybutynin in 358 subjects with urgency or urge incontinence, although there was no difference in clinical effect, there were fewer adverse events in the trospium group and better tolerability.[33] There are no CNS effects with this drug, which is especially important in the elderly.

Atropine

Atropine is rarely used in the treatment of DO because of its side-effects. Some trials have shown that intravesical atropine may have a benefit in women with neurogenic DO.[34]

Propantheline

Propantheline (Pro-Banthine) is a quaternary amine drug acting on both muscarinic and nicotinic acetylcholine receptors. It acts at the ganglionic level and at neuromuscular junctions. It is non-selective for muscarinic receptor subtypes and has a low, variable (5–10%) bioavailability. It is most effective when frequency of micturition is the major problem. The usual dose is 15–30 mg four times daily, but this is often ineffective and may need to be increased as high as 90 mg four times daily for benefit to be obtained. It is usually well tolerated with fewer side-effects than other agents, but is correspondingly less effective. It is not often used in clinical practice.

Musculotropic relaxants

These are direct-acting smooth muscle relaxants which also have anticholinergic actions. The group includes:

- oxybutynin chloride
- dicyclomine hydrochloride
- flavoxate hydrochloride.

Their side-effects are caused by their anti-cholinergic activity, which is often demonstrable at much lower doses than the muscle-relaxing effect. Among the drugs with mixed actions is terodiline, which was

withdrawn from the market as it was suspected of causing cardiac arrhythmias (*torsade de points*) in some subjects.

Smooth-muscle relaxants include:
- oxybutynin chloride
- dicyclomine hydrochloride
- flavoxate hydrochloride

Oxybutynin

For many years, the most effective and most commonly prescribed of these drugs was oxybutynin (which has been available in the UK since 1989). Particularly useful for those whose main complaint is urgency and urge incontinence, it unfortunately causes quite marked anticholinergic side-effects, as this is thought to be the main mode of action when given systemically. *In vitro*, the anticholinergic effect is 500 times stronger than the muscle-relaxing effect.[35] The commonest complaint is of dry mouth, reported by 87% of users (46% described it moderate or severe),[36] with cessation of treatment occurring in up to 37%.[37] Discontinuation is less likely if treatment is started at a low dose, and increased to the maximum therapeutic dose slowly over several weeks. It must be stressed to the patient that this is not merely a course of treatment, but that therapy might need to be life-long.

Oxybutynin is commonly prescribed for women who complain of urgency and urge incontinence

Due to its rapid onset of action and short half-life, oxybutynin may be taken on an as-required basis, for example before a long car journey, or before going shopping. This gives the patient some control over her condition and improves compliance.[37]

Oxybutynin can be taken on an 'as-needed' basis, which gives the patient some control over her condition and can improve compliance

Oxybutynin is a tertiary amine that shows high affinity for muscarinic M1 and M3 receptors, rather than M2. [M3 receptors are important mediators of bladder constriction. The bladder contains M2 and M3 receptors but the rule of M2 is unclear. M1 receptors are found outside the bladder.] It undergoes extensive first pass metabolism, and therefore has a low (6%) bioavailability. The metabolite, N-desethyl-oxybutynin, shows similar pharmacotherapeutic effects, although it occurs in much higher concentrations. It crosses the blood–brain barrier and so causes side-effects (nausea, dry mouth, constipation and CNS effects). This can therefore limit the therapeutic value due to dose limitation.

In addition to its antimuscarinic and muscle-relaxing activity, oxybutynin appears to have some local anaesthetic properties. This is probably only relevant in intravesical administration. Intravesical administration allows effective absorption from the bladder, with serum concentrations at least as high as with oral administration. Elimination is protracted, with oxybutynin and the metabolite (N-desethyloxybutynin) detectable even 24 hours post-dose in trials,[38] but the parent drug-to-metabolite ratio is much higher (1:2) than for oral preparations (1:10).

Oxybutynin has a well-documented efficacy in the treatment of DO, and is becoming more widely available with new and novel delivery systems. Together with tolterodine, it should be the first drug of choice for women with DO.[34]

> Women with DO should initially be given either oxybutynin or tolterodine to treat their symptoms

Propiverine

Propiverine has a documented beneficial effect in the treatment of DO and seems to have an acceptable side-effect profile.[39] It has combined anticholinergic and calcium-channel blocking actions, and although it is rapidly absorbed it undergoes extensive first-pass metabolism to several metabolites of uncertain pharmaco-

logical activity. The commonest side-effects are:

- dry mouth
- hypotension
- tiredness
- blurred vision in young people.

Although infrequently used in the UK, it is commonly prescribed in other parts of the world.

Flavoxate

The basis of the effect of flavoxate on the bladder has not been fully elucidated. It has been shown to:

- possess moderate calcium-antagonizing ability
- inhibit phosphodiesterase
- have some local anaesthetic action.

It has no anticholinergic action.[40] Investigators have failed to demonstrate any benefit over placebo.[41]

Tricyclic antidepressants

Imipramine, a tricyclic antidepressant, has complex pharmacological actions, including antimuscarinic activity, and serotonin and noradrenaline reuptake inhibition. Its exact mode of action in DO is not clear. However, the potentiation of serotonin and noradrenaline leads to detrusor relaxation and increased bladder outflow resistance. Combination of imipramine with propantheline has been shown to improve the clinical benefits.[42] It has been known for a long time that imipramine has favourable effects in the treatment of nocturnal enuresis in children.[43] However, even if it is generally considered that imipramine is a useful drug in the management of DO, there are no good randomized controlled trials to support its use.

There is limited experience with amitriptyline use for urgency–frequency syndromes and bladder pain.[44] Twenty-two subjects (12 male and 10 female) without interstitial cystitis and having vague non-specific urinary and pelvic or genital complaints were reviewed. All were treated with amitriptyline in doses ranging from 25–100 mg daily. Eleven subjects became symptom-free, six showed significant improvement and five did not respond. Fifteen subjects attempted tapering off the medication after six months, and 11 of these experienced an early return of symptoms. A therapeutic response was again seen with retreatment.

Therapeutic doses of tricyclic antidepressants may have serious toxic cardiac effects, especially in children, and can cause falls in the elderly.

> Therapeutic doses of tricyclic antidepressants can have serious toxic cardiac effects (particularly in children) and may cause falls in the elderly

Novel delivery systems

The advantages and disadvantages of novel delivery systems are listed in Table 6.3.

Extended-release oxybutynin

Extended-release preparations of oxybutynin (oxybutynin ER) have been developed. They utilize a novel delivery system that releases the drug at a constant rate over 24 hours. This avoids the peaks and troughs that are associated with the immediate-release versions.

In a multicentre comparison of extended-release versus immediate-release (IR) oxybutynin, although there was a similar reduction in urge incontinence episodes, there was a significant reduction in severe dry mouth symptoms (ER 25% vs IR 46%; $p=0.03$).[45] Oxybutynin ER (10 mg/day) was compared with tolterodine (2 mg bd) in a 12-week, randomized, double-blind, parallel-group study, involving 378 women with overactive bladder and known to be responsive to anticholinergics.[46] After 12 weeks and adjusting for baseline, oxybutynin ER was found to be significantly more effective than tolterodine in reducing:

- incontinence episode frequency
- frequency of micturition
- total incontinence.

> Extended-release oxybutinin releases the drug at a stable rate and avoids the' peaks and troughs' associated with the immediate-release preparation

The rates of dry mouth and other adverse effects were similar in both groups.

Transdermal oxybutynin has been investigated in a general population of subjects with overactive bladder and urge or mixed UI.[47] A total of 520 adult subjects were randomized to 12 weeks of double-blind daily treatment with oxybutynin transdermal delivery system (TDS) or placebo administered twice weekly. This was followed by a 12-week open-label, dose titration period. Doses of 2.6 and 3.9 mg oxybutynin TDS daily improved overactive bladder symptoms and quality-of-life, and were well tolerated. The most common adverse event was application site pruritus (oxybutynin TDS 10.8–16.8%, placebo 6.1%). Dry mouth incidence was similar in both groups (7.0% vs 8.3%, p not significant).

Table 6.3
Advantages and disadvantages of novel drug delivery systems

	Advantages	Disadvantages
Extended-release (oral)	● Efficacy maintained ● Reduced side-effects ● Once-daily dose ● Good compliance	● Unsuitable for 'as-needed' use ● Limited dose flexibility
Transdermal	● Efficacy similar to extended-release oral preparations ● Lowest incidence of side-effects in trials	● Patch-site pruritis
Intravesical	● Increases bladder capacity ● Local anaesthetic effect ● Few side-effects	● Learn clean intermittent self-catheter-ization or indwelling catheter

Oxybutynin TDS has also been compared with tolterodine ER and placebo.[48] Oxybutynin TDS and tolterodine ER were found to be effective and comparable treatments for urge and mixed incontinence when compared with placebo. Patients in the tolterodine ER and placebo groups applied placebo patches – application site reactions were most common in the oxybutynin TDS group (14% vs 4.3% with placebo). However, 4.1% of patients taking oxybutynin TDS reported dry mouth (vs 1.7% placebo, p not significant) compared with 7.3% of patients in the tolterodine ER group (p=0.0379 when compared with placebo). Oxybutynin TDS has the lowest reported incidence of adverse anticholinergic side-effects from large multicentre trials. [48]

> Large multicentre trials have reported that Oxybutyinin TDS has the lowest reported incidence of adverse anticholinergic side-effects when compared to other oxybutynin delivery methods

Rectal preparations of oxybutynin are available, but are not widely used.

Antidiuretic drugs

Desmopressin (1-desamino-8-D-arginine vasopressin, DDAVP) is a long acting synthetic analogue of vasopressin. It is available as an intranasal spray and, more recently, as a tablet. Desmopressin has been shown to be effective in reducing nocturia in patients with multiple sclerosis[49] and in those with nocturia of polyuric origin.[50]

> Desmopressin has been shown to reduce nocturia in patients with multiple sclerosis and in patients with nocturia of polyuric origin

During desmopressin therapy, the number of nocturnal voids and the nocturnal urine output are significantly reduced. Patients benefit from a longer period of uninterrupted sleep before the first nighttime void when compared with placebo.[51] Recent studies have also demonstrated benefit in daytime urinary frequency and incontinence.[52]

Desmopressin has similar antidiuretic properties to vasopressin, and leads to a reduction in urine production. It has less effect on smooth muscle, causing fewer problems with hypertension, bronchospasm and intestinal colic. It has been shown to be safe for long-term use.[53] However, its main side-effects are hyponatraemia and fluid retention, with weight gain. These effects must be considered, especially prior to its use in the elderly.

> The main side-effects of desmopressin are hyponatraemia and fluid retention with weight gain

Newer agents

Solifenacin

Solifenacin is a new, bladder-selective, long-acting, once-daily muscarinic antagonist. In a phase IIIa placebo-controlled trial to assess 5 and 10 mg of solifenacin against placebo, both doses showed a significant improvement in symptoms when compared with placebo, although 5 mg showed a better efficacy/tolerability balance.[54]

Darifenacin

Developed initially as a treatment for both irritable bowel syndrome and DO, darifenacin is a highly selective M3 receptor antagonist currently under development and soon to be licensed. In a pilot study on women with DO, it was effective in reducing total number, amplitude, and duration of overactive bladder contractions.[55] It was also shown to be less effective than oxybutynin at reducing salivary flow.[56]

Capsaicin and resiniferatoxin

Intravesical instillation of capsaicin, a neurotoxin extracted from red chilli peppers,[57] has a significant effect over placebo in the treatment of neurogenic DO. It exerts a biphasic effect on sensory nerves, with initial excitation being followed by a long-lasting blockade of C-fibres, which are rendered resistant to natural stimuli.[58] Side-effects of intravesical capsaicin include discomfort and a burning sensation at the pubic/urethral level during the installation. Prior instillation of local anaesthetic gel does not negate the effects of the capsaicin. There have been no reported malignant changes after repeated instillations, even up to five years. Bladder afferent desensitization with capsaicin is promising in subjects with motor or sensory bladder dysfunction, although initial pungency might limit its use.[59] It is not in clinical use for idiopathic DO.

Resiniferatoxin is an analogue of capsaicin extracted from *Eurphorbia*, a cactus-like plant. When given intravesically, it is 1000 times more potent than capsaicin in stimulating bladder activity. It has been shown to have fewer side-effects than capsaicin with a demonstrable increase in bladder capacity in up to 30% of subjects with DO.[60] Other studies, however, show little effect.[61]

> New drugs for the treatment of DO include solifenacin, darifenacin, capsaicin and resiniferatoxin

Surgical management

Conventional urogynaecological surgery is used for USI – it is unhelpful for DO and indeed may make matters worse. Many different surgical treatments have been tried over the years in the management of DO, but few are still in regular use today. Procedures long since abandoned include:

- bladder distension
- vaginal denervation
- bladder transection
- sacral neurectomy.

Their demise was caused by an unacceptably high rate of complications and limited efficacy.

Botulinum toxin A

Back in 1817 an illness caused by *Clostridium botulinum* toxin was first recorded – Justinus Kerner described a link between a sausage and a paralytic illness that affected 230 people. He was a district health officer and made botulism (Latin *botulus* meaning sausage) a notifiable disease.[62] In 1897, the microbiologist Emile-Pierre van Ermengen identified a Gram-positive, spore-forming, anaerobic bacterium in a ham that caused 23 cases of botulism in a Belgian nightclub. He termed the bacterium *Bacillus botulinus*. It was later re-termed *Clostridium botulinum*.[63] The discovery that botulinum toxin (Botox) blocks neuromuscular transmission and thereby causes weakness laid the foundations for its therapeutic development. In 1981 Alan Scott, an ophthalmologist, pioneered Botox therapy by using it to treat strabismus.[64]

The bacterium causes its effect by production of a neurotoxin. Different strains produce seven distinct serotypes designated A–G. All seven have a similar structure and molecular weight, consisting of a heavy (H) chain and a light (L) chain, joined by a disulphide bond.[65] They interfere with neural transmission by blocking the calcium-dependent release of the neurotransmitter acetylcholine, thereby causing the affected muscle to become weak and atrophic. The affected nerves do not degenerate, but as the blockage is irreversible, only the development of new nerve terminals and synaptic contacts allows recovery of function. This usually takes around three months.

> Botox has been effectively used to overcome outflow obstruction in women with voiding difficulty and to treat detrusor–sphincter dyssynergia after spinal cord injury

Despite the expense of repeated injections, in urogynaecology, Botox has been successfully used to overcome outflow obstruction in women with voiding difficulty[66] and to overcome detrusor–sphincter dyssynergia after spinal cord injury.[67, 68] It is currently the subject of research to assess its efficacy in the suppression of DO, although the long-term effects of repeated cystoscopic injections are not known.

Sacral neuromodulation

Electrical stimulation has been used in the management of both incontinence and voiding difficulty since 1963, but Tanagho and Schmidt first described implantable generators in 1981.

Stimulation of the S3 nerve root by an implanted electrical pulse generator can provide effective relief from frequency–urgency symptoms. In a prospective randomized trial of sacral neuromodulation versus delay, incontinence episode frequency (IEF), severity and pad use were all reduced in the active arm ($p<0.0001$). The results showed that 47% were dry and 29% reported a reduction in IEF of more than 50% at six months.[69] It is, however, very expensive as the implant alone costs around £10 000. Women need expert assessment, and management – although it is not suitable for routine use, sacral neuromodulation appears to be beneficial for a selected minority.

> Sacral neuromudulation is a very expensive treatment – the implant alone costs approximately £10 000

Prospective recipients are assessed in the first instance by temporary (external) stimulation, which, if helpful, progresses to implantation of a permanent stimulator.[70] The stimulator is a small electrical pulse generator, approximately the same size as a cardiac pacemaker, and is commonly implanted in the upper outer quadrant of the buttock. Complications most commonly reported are generator-site pain (15.9%) and implant-site pain (19.1%). Lead migration may occur in up to 7% of cases. The surgical revision of technical failures and complications was 32.5%.[69] This may be expected to reduce in the future as the technological development of generators and implants progresses.

Detrusor myectomy

Also known as auto-augmentation, the removal of the detrusor muscle allows the bladder mucosa to form a pseudodiverticulum. Large segments of muscle must be removed.[71] Although high cure rates of up to 80% are quoted for women with neurogenic DO,[72] it is more successful in women with idiopathic DO, and is associated with a gradual reduction in bladder capacity over time.

Augmentation cystoplasty

Augmentation cystoplasty is used to increase the size of the urinary reservoir. It is indicated in women who:

- lack adequate bladder capacity or detrusor compliance
- manifest debilitating frequency–urgency symptoms, with urge incontinence, recurrent UTIs or renal insufficiency
- have failed to derive benefit from medical therapy
- have a lifestyle that is severely limited
- have high-pressure urine storage endangering the upper renal tracts.

'Clam' cystoplasty

The operation most frequently used is the 'clam' cystoplasty. This involves bisecting the bladder, usually in the coronal plane anterior to the ureteric orifices, to within 1 cm of the bladder neck. A length of ileum is isolated and opened along its antemesenteric border. It is then sutured onto the defect in the bladder as a 'patch'. The ileal patch is thought to affect detrusor contractility and reduce the severity of DO by acting as an inert segment, absorbing overactive detrusor contractions.

> The most frequently used surgical procedure is 'clam' cystoplasty

A cure rate of up to 90% has been reported[73] when compared with Ingelman–Sundberg bladder denervation (54% complete response at

44 months)[74] and detrusor myectomy (63% showed improvement of compliance and/or resolution of detrusor contractions),[74] but the likelihood of early and late complications is also highest.

Postoperative complications

Postoperative complications include a significant risk of postoperative voiding difficulty, presumably secondary to a failure to generate adequate voiding pressures. This may be overcome by teaching the patient clean intermittent self-catheterization. Mucus production by the ileal segment may cause distress, especially when it is passed per urethram. This may be ameliorated by the ingestion of cranberry juice, which decreases mucus viscosity.[75]

Additionally there is an increased risk of urolithiasis. Of those who develop stones, there is a 30% risk of further stone formation within two years.[76] Electrolyte and acid–base balance may become disturbed, resulting in a metabolic acidosis. Malignant change occasionally occurs within the ileal segment. The bowel segment used for the cystoplasty does not seem relevant, and the mortality, where it occurs, is significant – as high as 30%. In one study 13 of the 16 cases reported had tuberculosis or chronic cystitis as the primary indication for cystoplasty.[77] Urinary nitrites, produced by recurrent bacterial infection, may also contribute to the malignant risk. The carcinogenic effects of these and nitrosamines have been implicated in tumours of urinary conduits and those with uretero-sigmoidostomy.[76]

Urinary diversion

In some women the bladder becomes severely contracted due to long-term DO. In these cases, drug therapy and behaviour modification are of little or no benefit, and augmentation cystoplasty is inappropriate and technically difficult. The only relief for intractable DO of idiopathic or neurogenic origin may be from a urinary diversion procedure with an ileal conduit. It may be easier to manage a stoma than to constantly change and wash wet underwear and continence pads.

> In some women drug therapy and behaviour modification are of no benefit and augmentation cystoplasty is technically difficult; in these women relief of DO may be from a urinary diversion procedure with an ileal conduit

Summary

Detrusor overactivity is a common disorder affecting millions of women worldwide. It is an easy condition to diagnose, but rather more difficult to treat. Treatment remains unsatisfactory and involves behavioural modification and therapy, accompanied by anticholinergic medication. Highly selective compounds are under development, which will increase the therapeutic options available. Only when these have failed is surgical intervention considered – it is always a last resort.

References

1. Brown JS. OAB: broadening our understanding and impact. Key Issues in the Treatment of Overactive Bladder. Seminar Session, 32nd Annual Meeting of the ICS, 2002.

2. Castleden CM, Duffin HM, Asher MJ. Clinical and urodynamic studies in 100 elderly women. *Br Med J Clin Res Ed* 1981; **282**:1103–5.

3. Abrams P, Cardozo L, Fall M et al. The standardisation of terminology of lower urinary tract function: report from the Standardisation Sub-Committee of the International Continence Society. *Neurourol Urodyn* 2002; **21**:167–78.

4. Jarvis GT, Millar DR. Controlled trial of bladder drill for detrusor instability. *Br Med J* 1980; **281**:1322–3.

5. Berghmans LC, Hendriks HJ, De Bie RA et al. Conservative treatment of urge urinary incontinence in women: a systematic review of randomised clinical trials. *BJU Int* 2000; **85**: 254–63.

6. Kinder RB, Mundy AR. Patho-physiology of idiopathic detrusor instability and detrusor heperrflexia. An in vitro study of human detrusor muscle. *Br J Urol* 1987; **60**: 509–5.

7. Gosling GA, Gilpin SA, Dixon JS, Gilpin CJ. Decrease in the autonomic innervation of human detrusor muscle in outflow obstruction. *J Urol* 1986; **136**: 501–4.

8. Cardozo LD, Stanton SL, Williams JE. Detrusor instability following surgery for stress incontinence. *Br J Urol* 1979; **51**: 204–7.

9. Hilton P. Urinary incontinence during sexual intercourse. A common, but rarely volunteered, symptom. *Br J Obstet Gynaecol* 1990; **95**: 377.

10. Cardozo LD, Stanton SL. Genuine stress incontinence and detrusor instability: a clinical and urodynamic review of 200 cases. *Br J Obstet Gynaecol* 1980; **87**: 184–90.

11. Sand PK, Hill RC, Ostergard DR. Incontinence history as a predictor of detrusor instability. *Obstet Gynaecol* 1988; **71**: 257–60.

12. Abrams P, Blaivas JG, Stanton SL, Andersen JT. The standardisation of terminology of lower urinary tract function. *Br J Obstet Gynaecol* 1990; **6(Suppl)**: 1–16.

13. Hosker G. Meeting of the ICS (UK), Leicester, April 2003.

14. Creighton SM, Stanton SL. Caffeine: does it affect your bladder? *Br J Urol* 1990; **66**: 613–14.

15. Jeffcoate TNA, Francis WJA. Urgency incontinence in the female. *Am J Obstet Gynaecol* 1966; **94**: 604–18.

16. Frewen WK. An objective assessment of the unstable bladder of psychological origin. *Br J Urol* 1978; **50**: 24–9.

17. Jarvis GJ, Millar DR. Controlled trial of bladder drill for detrusor instability. *Br Med J* 1980; **281**: 1322–3.

18. Wyman JF, Fantl JA, McClish DK *et al.* Quality of life following bladder training in older women with urinary incontinence. *Int J Pelvic Floor Dysfunct* 1997; **8**: 223–9.

19. Cardozo LD, Abrams P, Stanton SL, Fennelly RCL. Idiopathic detrusor instability treated by biofeedback. *Br J Urol* 1978; **50**: 24–9.

20. Cardozo LD, Stanton SL. Biofeedback – five year review. *Br J Urol* 1984; **56**: 220.

21. Plevnik S, Janez J, Vrtacnik P *et al.* Short term electrical stimulation: home treatment for urinary incontinence. *World J Urol* 1986; **4**: 24–6.

22. Freeman RM, Baxby K. Hypnotherapy for incontinence caused by the unstable bladder. *Br Med J* 1982; **284**: 1831–4.

23. Kelleher CJ, Filshie J, Khullar V, Cardozo LD. Acupuncture and the treatment of irritative bladder symptoms. *J Br Med Acupuncture Soc* 1994; **12**: 9–12.

24. Thuroff JW, Bunke B, Ebner A *et al.* Randomized, double-blind, multicenter trial on treatment of frequency, urgency and incontinence related to detrusor hyperactivity: oxybutynin versus propantheline versus placebo. *J Urol* 1991; **145**: 813–16.

25. Linjakumpu T, Hartikainen S, Klaukka T *et al.* Psychotropics among the home-dwelling elderly – increasing trends. *Int J Geriat Psych* 2002; **17(9)**: 874–83.

26. Stahl MMS, Ekström B, Sparf B *et al.* Urodynamic and other effects of tolterodine: a novel antimuscarinic drug for the treatment of DO. *Neurourol Urodyn* 1995; **14**: 647.

27. Brynne N, Stahl MMS, Hallén B. Pharmacokinetics and pharmacodynamics of tolterodine in man: a new drug for the treatment of urinary bladder overactivity. *Int J Clin Pharmacol Ther* 1997; **35**: 287.

28. Brynne N, Dalen P, Alvan G. Influence of CYP2D6 polymorphism on the pharmacokinetics and pharmacodynamics of tolterodine. *Clin Pharmacol Ther* 1998; **63**: 529–39.

29. Appell RA, Abrams P, Drutz HP *et al.* Treatment of overactive bladder: long-term tolerability and efficacy of tolterodine. *World J Urol* 2001; **19**: 141–7.

30. Van Kerrebroeck P, Kreder K, Jonas U *et al*; Tolterodine Study Group. Tolterodine once-daily: superior efficacy and tolerability in the treatment of the overactive bladder. *Urology* 2001; **57**: 414–21.

31. Abrams P, Freeman R, Anderstrom C *et al.* Tolterodine, a new anti-muscarinic agent: as effective but better tolerated than oxybutynin in women with an overactive bladder. *Br J Urol* 1998; **81**: 801–10.

32. Ückert S, Stief CG, Odenthal KP *et al.* Responses of isolated normal human detrusor muscle to various spasmolytic drugs commonly used in the treatment of the overactive bladder. *Arzneimittelforschung* 2000; **50**: 456.

33. Höfner K, Halaska M, Primus G *et al.* Tolerability and efficacy of trospium chloride in a long-term treatment (52 weeks) in women with urge-syndrome: a double-blind, controlled, multicentre clinical trial. *Neurourol Urodyn* 2000; **19**: 487.

34. Anderrson K-E *et al.* Pharmacological treatment of urinary incontinence. In: Abrams P, Cardozo LD, Khoury S, Wein A (eds). *Incontinence. 2nd International Consultation on Incontinence, July 1–3, 2001*. Health Publication, 2002, pp 479–511.

35. Kachur JF, Peterson JS, Carter JP *et al.* R and S enantiomers of oxybutynin: pharmacological effects in guinea pig bladder and intestine. *J Pharmacol Exp Ther* 1988; **247**: 867–72.

36. Anderson RU, Mobley D, Blank B *et al.* Once daily controlled versus immediate release oxybutynin chloride for urge urinary incontinence. OROS Oxybutynin study group. *J Urol* 1999; **161**: 1809–12.

37. Kelleher CJ, Cardozo LD, Khullar V *et al.* Anti-cholinergic therapy: the need for continued surveillance. *Neurourol Urodyn* 1994; **13**: 432–3.

38. Lehtoranta K, Tainio H, Lukkari-Lax E *et al.* Pharmacokinetics, efficacy, and safety of intravesical formulation of oxybutynin in women with DO. *Scand J Urol Nephrol* 2002; **36**: 18–24.

39. Madersbacher H, Halaska M, Voigt R *et al.* A placebo-controlled, multicentre study comparing the tolerability and efficacy of propiverine and oxybutynin in women with urgency and urge incontinence. *BJU Int* 1999; **84**: 646–51.

40. Guarneri L, Robinson E, Testa R. A review of flavoxate: pharmacology and mechanism of action. *Drugs Today* 1994; **30**: 91.

41. Chapple CR, Parkhouse H, Gardener C *et al.* Double-blind, placebo-controlled, cross-over study of flavoxate in the treatment of idiopathic detrusor instability. *Br J Urol* 1990; **66**: 491–4.

42. Raezer DM, Benson GS, Wein AJ, Duckett JW Jnr. The functional approach to the management of the pediatric neuropathic bladder: a clinical study. *J Urol* 1977; **177**: 649–54.

43. Hunsballe JM, Djurhuus JC. Clinical options for imipramine in the management of urinary incontinence. *Urol Res* 2001; **29**: 118–25.

44. Pranikoff K, Constantino G. The use of amitriptyline in women with urinary frequency and pain. *Urology* 1998; **51(Suppl 5A)**: 179–81.

45. Anderson RU, Mobley D, Blank B et al. Once daily controlled versus immediate release oxybutynin chloride for urge urinary incontinence. OROS Oxybutynin Study Group. *J Urol* 1999; **161**: 1809–12.

46. Appell RA, Sand P, Dmochowski R et al. Overactive Bladder: Judging Effective Control and Treatment Study Group. Prospective randomized controlled trial of extended-release oxybutynin chloride and tolterodine tartrate in the treatment of overactive bladder: results of the OBJECT Study. *Mayo Clin Proc* 2001; **76**: 358–63.

47. Dmochowski RR, Davila GW, Zinner NR et al, for The Transdermal Oxybutynin Study Group. Efficacy and safety of transdermal oxybutynin in women with urge and mixed urinary incontinence. *J Urol* 2002; **168**: 580–6.

48. Dmochowski RR, Sand PK, Zinner NR et al. Transdermal Oxybutynin Study Group. Comparative efficacy and safety of transdermal oxybutynin and oral tolterodine versus placebo in previously treated patients with urge and mixed urinary incontinence. *Urology* 2003; **62**: 237–42.

49. Hilton P, Hertogs K, Stanton SL. The use of desmopressin (DDAVP) for nocturia in women with multiple sclerosis. *J Neurol Neurosurg Psychiatry* 1983; **46**: 854–5.

50. Lose G, Lalos O, Freeman RM, van Kerrebroeck P; Nocturia study group. Efficacy of desmopressin (Minirin) in the treatment of nocturia: a double-blind placebo-controlled study in women. *Am J Obstet Gynecol* 2003; **189**: 1106–13.

51. Abrams P, Mattiasson A, Lose GR, Robertson GL. The role of desmopressin in the treatment of adult nocturia. *BJU Int* 2002; **90(Suppl 3)**: 32–6.

52. Robinson D, Cardozo L, Akeson M et al. Women take control; desmopressin – a drug for daytime urinary incontinence. *Neurourol Urodyn* 2002; **21**: 385–6.

53. Knudsen WB, Rittig S, Pedersen JB et al. Long-term treatment of nocturnal enuresis with desmopressin – influence on urinary output and haematological parameters. *Neurourol Urodyn* 1989; **8**: 348–9.

54. Cardozo LD. YM905: results of a randomised placebo-controlled trial in women with symptomatic overactive bladder. 18th Congress of the European Association of Urology. March 2003.

55. Rosario DJ, Leaker BR, Smith DJ et al. A pilot study of the effects of mutiple doses of the M3 muscarinic receptor antagonist darifenacin on ambulatory parameters of detrusor activity in women with detrusor instability. *Neurourol Urodyn* 1995; **14**: 464.

56. Mundy AR, Abrams P, Chapple CR et al. Darifenacin, the first selective M3 antagonist for overactive bladder: comparison with oxybutynin on ambulatory urodynamic monitoring and salivary flow. International Continence Society, 2001.

57. de Seze M, Wiart L, Joseph PA et al. Capsaicin and neurogenic detrusor hyperreflexia: a double-blind placebo-controlled study in 20 women with spinal cord lesions. *Neurourol Urodyn* 1998; **17**: 513–23.

58. Maggi CA. The dual, sensory and 'efferent' function of the capsaicin-sensitive primary sensory neurons in the urinary bladder and urethra. In Maggi CA (ed). *The Autonomic Nervous System, Volume 3, Nervous Control of the Urogenital System*. Chur: Harwood Academic Publishers, 1993, pp 383–422.

59. Cruz F, Guimaraes M, Silva C et al. Desensitization of bladder sensory fibers by intravesical capsaicin has long lasting clinical and urodynamic effects in women with hyperactive or hypersensitive bladder dysfunction. *J Urol* 1997; **157**: 585–9.

60. Lazzeri M, Beneforti P, Turini D. Urodynamic effects of intra-vesical resiniferatoxin in humans: preliminary results in stable and unstable detrusor. *J Urol* 1997; **158** 2093–7.

61. Cruz F, Guimaraes M, Silva C, Reis M. Suppression of bladder hyperreflexia by intravesical resiniferatoxin. *Lancet* 1997; **350**: 640–1.

62. Kerner J. Vergiftung durch verdobene Würste. *Tübinger Blätt Naturwißenschaften Arzenykunde* 1817; **3**: 1–25.

63. van Ermenegen E. Über einen neuen anaeroben Bacillus und seine Beziehungen zum Botulismus. *Z Hyg Infektionskrankh* 1897; **26**: 1–56.

64. Scott AB. Botulinum toxin injection of eye muscles to correct strabismus. *Trans Am Ophthalmol Soc* 1981; **79**: 734–70.

65. Dolly JO. Therapeutic and research exploitation of botulinum neurotoxins. *Eur J Neurol* 1997; **4(Suppl 2)**: S5–10.

66. Phelan MW, Franks M, Somogyi GT et al. Botulinum toxin urethral sphincter injection to restore bladder emptying in men and women with voiding dysfunction. *J Urol* 200; **165**: 1107–10.

67. Gallien P, Robineau S, Verin M et al. Treatment of detrusor sphincter dyssynergia by transperineal injection of botulinum toxin. *Arch Phys Med Rehabil* 1998; **79**: 715–17.

68. Schurch B, Hauri D, Rodic B et al. Botulinum-A toxin as a treatment of detrusor-sphincter dyssynergia: a prospective study in 24 spinal cord injury women. *J Urol* 1996; **155**: 1023–9.

69. Schmidt RA, Jonas U, Oleson KA et al. Sacral nerve stimulation for treatment of refractory urinary urge incontinence. Sacral Nerve Stimulation Study Group. *J Urol* 1999; **162**: 352–7

70. Janknegt RA, Weil EH, Eerdmans PH. Improving neuromodulation technique for refractory voiding dysfunctions: two-stage implant. *Urology* 1997; **49**: 358–62.

71. Daneshgari F, Dmochowski R, Ghoniem G *et al*. Surgical treatment of incontinence in women. In Abrams P, Cardozo LD, Khoury S, Wein A (eds). *Incontinence. 2nd International Consultation on Incontinence, July 1–3, 2001*. Health Publication, 2002, pp 825–63.

72. Swami SK, Abrams P, Hammonds JC *et al*. Treatment of DO with detrusor myectomy (bladder autoaugmentation). Presented at the 23rd Congress of the Societé Internationale d'Urologie 1994; abstract 580.

73. Mark SD, McRae CU, Arnold EP, Gowland SP. Clam cystoplasty for the overactive bladder: a review of 23 cases. *Aust NZ J Surg* 1994; **64**: 88–90.

74. Westney OL, McGuire EJ. Surgical procedures for the treatment of urge incontinence. *Tech Urol* 2001; **7**: 126–32.

75. Avorn J, Monane M, Gurnitz JH *et al*. Reduction of bacturia and pyuria after ingestion of cranberry juice. *JAMA* 1994; **271**: 751–4.

76. Gough DCS. Enterocystoplasty. *BJU Int* 2001; **88**: 739–43.

77. Fernandez-Arjona M, Herrerro L, Romera J *et al*. Synchronous signet ring cell carcinoma and squamous cell carcinoma arising in an augmented ileocystoplasty. Case report and review of the literature. *Eur Urol* 1996; **29**: 125–8.

7. Voiding difficulty

Definitions
Aetiology
Clinical features
Investigations
Treatment

Normal voiding occurs when the pelvic floor and urethral sphincter relax prior to a detrusor contraction. This mechanism is partly under conscious control from the brain, partly dependent on a sacral reflex arc and partly controlled by direct innervations of the bladder, sphincter and pelvic floor.

Voiding difficulty may be secondary to either a failure of detrusor function or to outflow obstruction. The two conditions can occur together. They represent a spectrum of conditions, ranging from subclinical minor problems only diagnosed after urodynamics or ultrasound, to acute or chronic retention. Voiding difficulty in women is surprisingly common. In a study of 1193 consecutive women referred for urodynamic investigation, Dwyer et al found that 165 (13.8%) had some form of voiding dysfunction.[1] In 138 of these women the voiding difficulty was associated with detrusor overactivity (DO), urodynamic stress incontinence (USI) or bladder hypersensitivity.

> Voiding difficulty can be secondary to outflow obstruction or to a failure of detrusor function

Definitions

Acute retention is the painful percussable or palpable bladder when the patient is unable to pass any urine.[2] There are, however, occasions when it may be painless, such as after epidural anaesthesia,[3] or associated with a prolapsed intervertebral disc.[2] Chronic retention of urine is a non-painful bladder, palpable after the patient has passed urine. Such patients may be incontinent.[2]

Aetiology

Pharmacological causes

The commonest pharmacological cause of acute retention in women is obstetric epidural use. Sadly, the catastrophic damage to the bladder resulting from overdistension is also easily preventable.[4]

> The most common pharmacological cause of acute retention in women is obstetric epidural use

Drugs that interfere with the function of cholinergic synapses can theoretically cause voiding difficulty. Anticholinergic agents and antimuscarinic agents, used in the management of DO, should be prescribed with care if there appears to be any problem with bladder emptying at urodynamics. However, a small study performed at King's College Hospital showed that in women with mild voiding difficulty there did not appear to be any worsening of problems when these drugs were taken.[5]

Obstructive causes

Outflow obstruction in the form of prostatic enlargement is a frequent cause of voiding difficulty in men. Obstructive voiding is infrequently diagnosed in women.[6] Previous incontinence surgery and severe urogenital prolapse are the commonest causes, accounting for around one-half of cases.[7] Urethral stricture, which may be caused by chronic inflammation or atrophy, accounts for only 13% of cases.

> In women, previous incontinence surgery and severe urogenital prolapse are the most common obstructive causes of voiding difficulty

Extrinsic pressure from a posterior fibroid, classically in association with a gravid uterus, is an infrequent but well described cause of urinary retention. It may also be seen with compression from other pelvic masses or faecal impaction. Foreign bodies and bladder stones are very rare.

Inflammatory causes

It is well known that any condition causing pain in the vagina or urethra can be associated with urinary retention. Postoperative recovery is frequently complicated by urinary retention, and catheterization should be undertaken to relieve it. Inflammation may also occur with other chemical or allergic irritants. Active vulval herpes may act as a vulval irritant causing inflammation, but may also result in lumbosacral meningomyelitis, therefore being a central cause of acute retention.[3]

Detrusor failure

Overflow incontinence occurs when the bladder, secondary to an injury or insult, becomes large and flaccid, with little or no detrusor tone or function. Ischaemic damage to the bladder causes inflammation and healing by deposition of scar tissue. The result is a permanent loss of function.

> If the detrusor muscle loses tone and function, overflow incontinence occurs, and a permanent loss of function results

Diagnosis

The condition is diagnosed when the urinary residual is more than 50% of the bladder capacity. The bladder simply leaks as it becomes full – the sequelae of this are:

- reduced functional capacity
- reduced frequency of micturition
- recurrent urinary tract infection.

In the longer term, there may be hydroureter, hydronephrosis and chronic renal failure secondary to reflux nephropathy.

Fowler syndrome

There are a number of women who develop acute retention on several occasions, usually after a minor stimulus. Fowler and Kirby have described a primary disorder of the urethral sphincter.[8] The sphincter becomes hypertrophied and fails to relax. The diagnosis is highly specialized, using an electron micrograph of the sphincter, where characteristic 'whale noises' are described. There may be an association with polycystic ovarian syndrome.

Spinal problems

Cauda equina syndrome results from compression of the cauda equina by a space-occupying lesion in the spinal canal (eg a protruding disc) below the level of L2. It is a severe neurological deficit, and presents with:

- low back pain
- motor weakness
- sensory deficit in the sacral area
- voiding difficulty or urinary incontinence.

It is an absolute indication for acute surgical decompression of lumbar disc herniation.

> Patients with cauda equina syndrome present with voiding difficulty or urinary incontinence, motor weakness, sensory deficit in the sacral area, and low back pain. It is an indication for acute surgical decompression of lumbar disc herniation

Meta-analysis has shown that preoperative chronic lower back pain or preoperative rectal dysfunction carries a worse prognosis for resolution of urinary incontinence.[9] Outcome overall is improved in those decompressed within 48 hours.

Multiple sclerosis

Bladder dysfunction is seen in up to 75% of multiple sclerosis (MS) sufferers. Patients present with symptoms of urgency, frequency and urge incontinence.[10] The commonest abnormality is DO, although detrusor–sphincter dyssynergia may produce an interrupted flow pattern and incomplete emptying.

> Up to 75% of multiple sclerosis sufferers have bladder dysfunction, with detrusor overactivity being the commonest defect

In their review article, DasGupta and Fowler argue that in a known case of MS, cystometry is unnecessary for the investigation of bladder symptoms as the underlying mechanism can be presumed to be DO.[10] Treatment should be aimed at the DO using the same drugs as in non-neurogenic patients. Desmopressin (as Desmospray) is licensed for the treatment of nocturia in MS where other therapies have failed. It is important, however, to limit fluid intake in case of hyponatraemia.

Where the residual volume of urine exceeds ~100 ml, it is important that the bladder is kept empty. This may be achieved either by the use of a permanent in-dwelling catheter or by the use of clean intermittent self-catheterization (CISC). Intravesical therapy can then also be initiated for the DO.

Clinical features

Some women may be asymptomatic and diagnosed fortuitously, but the majority of women with voiding difficulty present with:

- poor stream
- few voids
- a sense of incomplete emptying
- straining to void.

Others may present with overflow incontinence. Acute retention usually presents with pain and an inability to void.

Investigations

Frequency–volume chart

The woman should be encouraged to keep an accurate diary of her intake and output habits. Frequent micturition of small volumes with incontinence suggests overflow. Infrequent voiding may predispose to urinary tract infection.

Uroflowmetry

The woman should be encouraged to attend for uroflowmetry investigation with a comfortably full bladder. As a single measurement may be unreliable, she should be encouraged to sit normally on the commode, rather than hover, and repeat measurements should be taken in full privacy. Repeated flow rates below 15 ml per second, where the voided volume is greater than 150 ml, are suggestive of voiding difficulty.

> Repeated flow rates below 15 ml per second, where the voided volume is greater than 150 ml, are indicative of voiding difficulty

Cystometry

It is possible to record a normal flow rate in situations of mild outflow obstruction, because the detrusor has some reserve and may compensate. Subtracted cystometry will detect this. Additionally, subtracted cystometry will differentiate between outflow obstruction (high detrusor pressure, low flow) and detrusor failure (low detrusor pressure, low flow).

Urethral pressure profilometry

The role of tests of urethral function remains controversial, but urethral pressure profilometry is useful for identifying a possible urethral stricture. Urethral closure pressure declines with advancing age, and so an unusually high closure pressure, combined with pressure–flow evidence of outflow obstruction, is highly suggestive of stricture.

> Urethral pressure profilometry is useful for identifying possible urethral stricture

Radiographic imaging

An X-ray of the lumbar spine and sacrum may be indicated where other tests have failed to identify a cause. Narrowing of the disc space may indicate a disc problem, which can be further investigated by magnetic resonance imaging (MRI). Ultrasound, intravenous urography or MRI may also be useful to investigate pelvic masses causing outflow obstruction.

> Ultrasound, intravenous urography and MRI are useful to investigate pelvic masses that may be causing outflow obstruction

Treatment

Behavioural modification

Mild cases of voiding difficulty may require no treatment. Drugs with anticholinergic side-effects should be withdrawn where possible, and frequency or urinary tract infection secondary to chronic residual should be alleviated by double voiding. (This is where after a 'normal' void the woman goes back to the toilet after a few minutes to void again.)

In cases of voiding difficulty following incontinence surgery a change in position may be helpful. The angle of the urethra is often changed, and so a more upright posture whilst voiding may aid emptying.

Some women with mild voiding difficulty only complain of nocturia. This occurs because they void off the top of a chronic residual, which reduces the functional bladder capacity. Reducing the fluid intake in the evenings, and avoiding caffeine or alcohol, may be all that is required.

Catheterization

In the event of an acute urinary retention and distension injury, the bladder should be rested. This is best achieved by free catheter drainage, perhaps for a few weeks. Therefore, a supra-pubic catheter is preferable, both for ease of management and comfort and as they are associated with a lower risk of infection. Supra-pubic catheters are easily inserted. It is a day-case procedure conducted under regional or general anaesthetic. The catheter can be clamped to allow urethral voiding and thereafter check the residual volume. This is part of the rehabilitation of the bladder

> Suprapubic catheters are associated with a low risk of infections, are easy to insert and manage, and are relatively comfortable

Where possible, it is preferable to teach the woman CISC. This method is associated with lower rates of urinary tract infection than long-term indwelling catheters.[11] Although motivation and manual dexterity are a prerequisite, in a descriptive study of 163 patients of both sexes, 140 found the technique easy or very easy.[12] The frequency of CISC is determined on the basis of the residual volumes – when the residual is consistently less than 100–150 ml, it can be stopped.

Surgery

Adequate and appropriate investigation may reveal a pelvic mass as the cause of voiding difficulty. Surgical removal of a fibroid uterus or a large ovarian cyst may be appropriate.

Where investigations have shown evidence of urethral stricture, urethrotomy is preferable to urethral dilatation. Dilatation is associated with early failure, and subsequent dilatation may cause urethral fibrosis or damage to the urethral sphincter mechanism. Either an Otis urethrotomy or a cystoscopically guided urethrotomy is performed, with three incisions along the length of the urethra. A large bore catheter is left *in situ* for two weeks to allow healing and it is recommended to conduct CISC on a weekly basis to help maintain patency.

References

1. Dwyer PL, Desmedt E. Impaired bladder emptying in women. *Aust NZ J Obstet Gynaecol* 1994; **34**: 73–8.
2. Abrams P, Cardozo L, Fall M *et al*. The standardisation of terminology of lower urinary tract function: report from the Standardisation Sub-Committee of the International Continence Society. *Neurourol Urodyn* 2002; **21**: 167–78.

3. Monga AK. Non-neurogenic voiding difficulties and retention. In Staskin D, Cardozo LD (eds). *Textbook of Female Urology and Urogynaecology*. Oxford: Isis Medical Media 2001, pp 855–63.

4. Jackson SR, Barry C, Davies G *et al*. Length of labour and epidural anaesthesia: long term effects on urinary symptoms. *Int Urogynecol J* 1995; **6**: 244.

5. Robinson D, Dixon A, Cardozo L *et al*. Overactive bladder: does antimuscarininc therapy exacerbate significant voiding difficulties? 11th Annual ICS (UK) Annual Scientific Meeting, Bournemouth, March 2004: oral abstract 024.

6. Patel R, Nitti V. Bladder outlet obstruction in women: prevalence, recognition, and management. *Curr Urol Rep* 2001; **2**: 379–87.

7. Groutz A, Blaivas JG, Chaikin DC. Bladder outlet obstruction in women: definition and characteristics. *Neurourol Urodyn* 2000; **19**: 213–20.

8. Fowler CJ, Kirby RS. Abnormal electromyographic activity (decelerating burst and complex repetitive discharges) in the striated urethral sphincter in 5 women with urinary retention. *Br J Urol* 1985; **57**: 67–70.

9. Ahn UM, Ahn NU, Buchowski JM *et al*. Cauda equina syndrome secondary to lumbar disc hernaition: a meta-analysis of surgical outcomes. *Spine* 2000; **25**: 1515–22.

10. DasGupta R, Fowler CJ. Bladder, bowel and sexual dysfunction in multiple sclerosis: management strategies. *Drugs* 2003; **63**: 153–66.

11. Hunt GM, Whitaker RH, Doyle PT. Intermittent self catheterisation in adults. *Br Med J (Clin Res Ed)* 1984; **289**: 467–8.

12. Webb RJ, Lawson AL, Neal DE. Clean intermittent self-catheterisation in 172 adults. *Br J Urol* 1990; **65**: 20–3.

8. Recurrent urinary tract infection

Aetiology
Investigation
Treatment

Acute urinary tract infection (UTI) is very common. There are an estimated 0.5–0.7 episodes per person-year[1] among women, who are disproportionately affected. It is usually accepted that a pure culture of 10^5 organisms/ml urine, obtained from a mid-stream 'clean catch' specimen of urine, is diagnostic of infection.[2] Approximately 25% of women who have an episode of acute UTI go on to have recurrent episodes.[3] The occurrence of three or more confirmed UTIs in a one-year period constitutes recurrent UTI.

> 25% of women who have an episode of acute urinary tract infection go on to have recurrent episodes

Aetiology
Vaginal flora

Uropathic bacteria, most commonly *Escherichia coli*, enter the bladder from the vagina or perineum, but are expelled by voiding. Any process that impairs voiding function or voiding frequency may predispose to UTI.

> Three or more confirmed UTIs in one year constitures recurrent UTI

Uropathic bacteria tend to have fimbriae (as found on all *E. coli*), which allow initial adherence of the uropathogen to the mucosa. Compared with women without recurrent infection, those with such infections have longer durations of vaginal colonization with uropathic *E. coli* and threefold more *E. coli* adhering to vaginal, buccal and voided uroepithelial cells.[4]

The normal vaginal flora may be disrupted and predisposed to colonization with such uropathic organisms. Factors causing this include:

- recent use of β-lactam antibiotics[5]
- the postmenopausal state.[6]

Lack of oestrogen stimulation leads to a reduction in glycogen production – normal vaginal lactobacilli need glycogen for metabolism, and so colonization by uropathogens becomes easier. Atrophic urethritis and vaginitis in postmenopausal women is often associated with urinary tract symptoms. This is due to epithelial and submucosal thinning of the urethra, with consequential irritation and loss of the mucosal seal.[7]

> Colonization by uropathogens is easier when there is a lack of oestrogen, eg in postmenopausal women

Other causes

Oestrogen receptors have been identified in the brain, micturition centre, bladder, urethra and pelvic floor. The menopause, and subsequent oestrogen deficiency, has been implicated in the aetiology of recurrent UTI.[6]

Sexual activity and contraceptive diaphragm use predispose to UTI, and spermicidal lubricants increase this risk.[5] Many women dramatically reduce their fluid intake, either to ameliorate the effects of urinary incontinence or because of a hectic lifestyle. This causes infrequent voiding and stasis of urine in the bladder, which in turn predisposes to infection.

> Sexual activity and diaphragm use can predispose to urinary tract infection; spermicidal lubricants also increase this risk

Cystocele may cause 'kinking' of the urethra, analogous or a kinked garden hose that does not flow well. A large cystocele may act as a urinary 'sump' and allow urinary stasis. Rectocele and faecal impaction, especially in the elderly, may compress the urethra and cause outflow obstruction.

Investigation

It is logical that culture of a midstream specimen of urine should be tested, and treatment instituted according to the results. Intravenous urography is usually normal and is not recommended as a first-line investigation – at least not in the primary-care setting. Rather, ultrasound of the kidneys and X-ray of the kidneys, ureters and bladder reduces exposure to radiation and adequately investigates the upper renal tracts.

> Ultrasound of the kidneys and X-rays of the kidneys, ureters and bladder are the first-line method of investigation of the upper renal tracts

Cystourethroscopy

Cystourethroscopy is often performed in cases of recurrent UTI. In the elderly it is especially useful, as UTI may be the presenting symptom of tumour or calculus. Otherwise, it is useful to identify morphological abnormalities, such as diverticula. Bladder base biopsy in other groups normally reveals chronic inflammation, consistent with infection.

Urodynamics

Urodynamics in women with recurrent UTI who are below 40 years of age are usually normal. Urodynamics are strongly indicated in women with previous bladder-neck surgery, many of whom will be shown to have voiding difficulty secondary to outflow obstruction. Women with 'culture-negative' episodes of cystitis are often shown to have detrusor overactivity.

Treatment

General principles

Treatment should be aimed at relieving or removing the underlying cause of infection. Incomplete emptying should be investigated and treated to reduce or overcome outflow obstruction. This can be done surgically or by use of clean intermittent self-catheterization. Surgical repair of a cystocele may unkink the urethra and aid voiding; urethrotomy to a urethral stricture may overcome the limitation to flow.

> Treatment for UTI should be targeted to remove or relieve the underlying cause of infection

Women should be advised to maintain an adequate fluid intake of 1–1.5 litres per day, which allows for a reasonable urine production and output, without being excessive. Constipation and faecal impaction should be treated. At King's College we normally advise women to shower before intercourse and void afterwards. It is also appropriate to offer advice and review their method of contraception.

Antibiotics

Prophylactic use of antibiotics in recurrent UTI is limited. Continuous daily use or alternate-day use of an antibiotic has been advocated in acute UTI,[8] but the major concern is the development of resistant strains with consequent increased morbidity. The use of antibiotic prophylaxis should therefore be individualized. Continuous antibiotics are not indicated in women with in-dwelling catheters, as colonization still occurs and morbidity is not altered.

> Prophylactic use of antibiotics for UTI is limited. This is mainly because of the development of resistant strains, with consequent increased morbidity

Oestrogens

Oestrogen therapy has been shown to increase vaginal pH and reverse the microbiological changes that occur in the vagina following the menopause.[9]

A meta-analysis (conducted by the Hormones and Urogenital Therapy Committee) on data from 334 subjects in 10 studies revealed a significant benefit from oestrogen over placebo (odds ratio = 2.51, 95% confidence interval = 1.48–4.25).[10] Although a variety of different oestrogen preparations were used in the reports, vaginal administration seemed to be most effective in the prevention of recurrent UTI in postmenopausal women.

> Oestrogen therapy has been shown to raise vaginal pH and reverse the microbiological changes that occur in the vagina after the menopause

Cranberry juice

Cranberry juice contains fructose, which could interfere with the adhesion of the fimbriae of uropathic bacteria to the bladder mucosa.[11] A well-designed study has demonstrated a reduction in episodes of bacteriuria and pyuria in a population of 153 elderly women (mean age 78.5 years) who drink 300 ml of either cranberry juice or a placebo drink, per day.[12] Subjects randomized to the cranberry beverage had a risk of bacteriuria (defined as organisms numbering $\geq 10^5$ /ml) with pyuria that was only 42% of that in the control group ($p=0.004$). Their chance of remaining bacteruric–pyuric, given that they were bacteruric–pyuric in the previous month, was only 27% of the chance in the control group ($p=0.006$). Both cranberry tablets and cranberry juice have also been shown to reduce the risk of UTI in sexually active women (aged 21–72) experiencing at least one symptomatic UTI per year (to 20% and 18% respectively) compared with placebo (to 32%) ($p<0.05$).[13] Cost-effectiveness ratios revealed that cranberry tablets were twice as cost effective as organic cranberry juice.

> Cranberry, in juice or tablet form, is a safe, naturally occurring substance that has been demonstrated to reduce the risk of UTI in sexually active women

Bearing in mind the potential for side-effects and the likelihood of resistant bacteria in patients receiving conventional antibiotic prophylaxis, the opportunity of giving a safe, naturally occurring substance, such as cranberry juice, deserves further consideration.[14]

References

1. Hooton TM, Scholes D, Hughes JP et al. A prospective study of risk factors for urinary tract infection in young women. N Engl J Med 1996; 335: 468–74.

2. Kass EH. Bacteriuria and the diagnosis of infections of the urinary tract. AMA Arch Int Med 1957; 100: 709–14.

3. Foxman B. Recurring urinary tract infection: incidence and risk factors. Am J Public Health 1990; 80: 331–3.

4. Schaeffer AJ, Jones JM, Dunn JK. Association of in vitro Escherichia coli adherence to vaginal and buccal epithelial cells with susceptibility of women to recurrent urinary-tract infections. N Engl J Med 1981; 304: 1062–6.

5. Stapleton A. Prevention of recurrent urinary-tract infections in women. Lancet 1999; 353: 7–8.

6. Hextall A. Oestrogens and lower urinary tract function. Maturitas 2000; 36: 83–92.

7. Hextall A, Cardozo L. Managing postmenopausal cystitis. Hosp Pract (Office Edn) 1997; 32: 191–8.

8. Brumfitt W, Hamilton-Miller JMT. Efficacy and safety profile of longterm nitrofurantoin in urinary tract infection: 18 years' experience. J Antimicrob Chemother 1998; 42: 363–71.

9. Brandberg A, Mellstrom D, Samsioe G. Low dose oral oestriol treatment in elderly women with urogenital infections. Acta Obstet Gynaecol Scand 1987; 140: 33–8.

10. Cardozo L, Lose G, McClish D et al. A systematic review of estrogens for recurrent urinary tract infections: third report of the hormones and urogenital therapy (HUT) committee. Int Urogynecol J Pelvic Floor Dysfunct 2001; 12: 15–20.

11. Zafriri D, Ofek I, Adar R et al. Inhibitory activity of cranberry juice on adherence of type 1 and type P fimbriated Escherichia coli to eukaryotic cells. Antimicrob Ag Chemother 1989; 33: 92–8.

12. Avorn J, Monane M, Gurwitz JH et al. Reduction of bacteriuria an pyuria after ingestion of cranberry juice. JAMA 1994; 324: 751–4.

13. Stothers L. A randomized trial to evaluate effectiveness and cost effectiveness of naturopathic cranberry products as prophylaxis against urinary tract infection in women. Can J Urol 2002; 9: 1558–62.

14. Kerr KG. Cranberry juice and prevention of recurrent urinary tract infection. Lancet 1999; 353: 673.

9. Other lower urinary tract disorders

Frequency–urgency and painful bladder syndromes
Interstitial cystitis
Sensory urgency
Urethral problems

Numerous conditions can affect the bladder without causing incontinence. Careful investigation is required to identify the underlying aetiology as the treatments are very different. Some conditions, such as a urinary tract infection (UTI) or poor habit, are easily rectified. Some of the other causes tend to run a chronic course and include a number of very disabling conditions.

Frequency–urgency and painful bladder syndromes

These are common urinary symptoms in women. They can be very distressing and have been shown to cause a major adverse effect on social function and quality-of-life. Overactive bladder syndrome (OAB) is the combination of frequency and urgency, with or without urge incontinence, and nocturia. Quality-of-life scores for women suffering from these sensory symptoms have been shown to be worse than those complaining of other urinary symptoms, including incontinence.[1] The combination of irritative bladder symptoms (frequency, urgency, nocturia and dysuria) with pain and negative urine cultures gives rise to an ill-defined group of conditions known as 'painful bladder syndromes'. In the majority of cases the exact pathogenesis is uncertain and available treatments are largely empirical.

> Overactive bladder syndrome (OAB) is the combination of frequency and urgency (with or without urge incontinence), and nocturia

Incidence

Epidemiological data suggests that up to 20% of women complain of frequency and around 15% complain of urgency.[2] These figures increase only slightly with age. Associated pain on bladder filling or on micturition is a less common but highly disabling symptom.

Aetiology

There are a large number of disorders in the lower urinary tract, and further afield, that can cause these symptoms. Listed in Table 9.1 are

Table 9.1
Conditions causing frequency–urgency, with or without pain

Arising from the lower urinary tract	*Outside the lower urinary tract*
● Detrusor overactivity	● Excessive fluid intake
● Urinary tract infection	● Maladaptive learned behaviour
● Functionally small bladder	● Diuretic drugs
● Radiation cystitis	● Congestive cardiac failure
● Chronic urinary residual	● Pelvic mass
● Cystocele	● Diabetes mellitus
● Oestrogen deficiency	● Diabetes insipidus
● Bladder calculus	● Upper motor neurone lesion
● Bladder tumour	● Renal disease
● Interstitial cystitis	● Pregnancy
● Sensory urgency	
● Urethritis	
● Detrusor hyperreflexia secondary to neurological damage	

some of the most common causes. A number of these conditions are mentioned elsewhere in this book. The group of conditions that cause bladder pain in association with frequency and urgency are considered below. This is a poorly defined collection of diseases – considered a spectrum of 'painful bladder syndromes' – that may share a common aetiology. Exact classification is hampered by:

- the lack of universally agreed definitions
- poor understanding of the pathogenesis of these conditions
- the absence of robust research evidence on which to base treatment.

Management

History

Patients presenting with frequency–urgency need to be carefully questioned about associated urinary symptoms. Associated urge incontinence and its severity is important, as is any associated dysuria or suprapubic pain. If haematuria is reported then this must be investigated further. The presence of the following need to be excluded:

- urinary tract infection
- bladder carcinoma
- calculus
- lesion of the upper urinary tracts.

Patients presenting with frequncy–urgency need to have the following conditions ruled out:
- urinary tract infection
- bladder carcinoma
- calculus
- lesion of the upper urinary tracts

As there is such a wide-ranging differential diagnosis for possible causes of urinary frequency–urgency, conditions both within the urinary tract and further afield need to be considered. Information should be sought regarding any neurological symptoms, drinking habits and concomitant medication.

Examination

An abdominal examination will rule out a mass or large distended bladder. A neurological assessment is important to exclude an upper motor neurone lesion. The S2, S3 and S4 nerve roots innervate the bladder, and particular regard should be paid to these dermatomes.

Abdominal examination should rule out a mass or large distended bladder, and neurological assessment should exclude upper motor neurone lesions

On pelvic examination a possible large fibroid uterus, ovarian mass or pregnancy should be considered. It is important to assess the degree and site of any pelvic organ prolapse that may be present. Tenderness on bladder palpation may be found in interstitial cystitis (IC) and other painful bladder syndromes. The urethra should be carefully inspected for a local cause (such as a urethral caruncle) of irritative symptoms, or signs of urethritis.

Investigations

Investigations are described in more detail in Chapter 3.

Initial investigation should always include a midstream urine sample for culture and sensitivity and urine for cytology. Appropriate cultures may be indicated for:

- 'fastidious organisms' (*Mycoplasma hominis, Ureaplasma urealyticum, Chlamydia trachomatis*)
- tuberculosis
- schistosomiasis.

A completed frequency–volume chart is an invaluable tool, providing useful information on fluid input and output, drinking habits, voided volumes and the episodes of urgency and incontinence.

Where the cause for the symptoms is not revealed by the above assessment, the more specialist investigations should be considered. Ultrasound scan can be accurately used to assess urinary residual volumes, to measure bladder wall thickness and to give more information on any masses detected on pelvic examination. Once a UTI has been ruled out, subtracted cystometry may detect detrusor overactivity (DO) or sensory urgency. Cystourethroscopy should be performed for recurrent UTI if haematuria is present, if pain is a significant symptom and if IC or a urethral diverticulum is suspected. This can be undertaken with:

- a flexible cystoscope under local anaesthetic
- a rigid cystoscope under general anaesthetic.

> Specialist investigations are only recommended if standard assessment fails to indicate a cause of the frequency–urgency symptoms

The latter is more common and allows far better biopsy samples to be taken for histological assessment, which is important in the diagnosis of many of these conditions. Although the histological appearances of biopsies taken from patients with IC are generally non-specific, the findings at cystoscopy are more characteristic.

Treatment

Treatment should be directed at the underlying cause of the urinary symptoms. This intervention is supported by evidence, such as a simple course of antibiotics for a UTI, or bladder retraining and anticholinergic drug therapy for DO. With some of the less well-understood or rarer diseases, treatment may be largely empirical with less chance of success. This is often the case in women with IC.

Bladder retraining is widely used to treat many of the disorders giving rise to symptoms of urinary frequency–urgency, including DO and sensory urgency. The patient is taught to slowly increase the interval between voiding episodes so that frequency can be reduced and the functional cystometric capacity increases. This

technique was used by Jarvis to treat women with sensory urgency. He demonstrated that >50% of these women were symptom-free and objectively dry six months after treatment with bladder retraining.[3]

> Bladder retraining is commonly used to treat many of the disorders that cause symptoms of urinary frequency–urgency, including detrusor overactivity and sensory urgency

Interstitial cystitis

This chronic inflammatory disorder of the bladder is notoriously difficult to manage and can result in considerable morbidity. Quality-of-life scores in women with IC are consistently low. Women between the ages of 40 and 60 years are most commonly affected. The condition occurs far more frequently in Caucasians and there is a 9:1 female predominance.[4] Reported prevalence rates for this condition vary widely as there is no universally accepted definition.

> Interstitial cystitis is most common in women aged between 40 and 60

Aetiology

The aetiology remains obscure but the following have all been postulated:

- infection
- autoimmune disease
- epithelial cell dysfunction
- allergy
- psychosomatic disorder
- an inability to repair the normal protective layer of glycosaminoglycans.

The diagnosis of IC is based on suggestive symptoms and characteristic cystoscopy findings. Typical symptoms include:

- frequency
- urgency

- dysuria
- pain (in the absence of bacterial cystitis)
  - lower abdominal
  - bladder
  - vaginal
  - urethral
  - perineal.

> Diagnosis of interstitial cystitis is based on suggestive symptoms (eg frequency, pain, urgency and dysuria) and characteristic cystoscopic findings (eg subepithelial petechial haemorrhages, splotchy haemorrhages, linear cracking of the mucosa, white urothelial scars and ulceration)

Voiding often relieves the suprapubic discomfort, and drinking alcohol and caffeine-containing drinks frequently exacerbates the pain. In an attempt to standardize diagnosis, the National Institute of Arthritis, Diabetes, Digestive and Kidney Diseases published consensus criteria in 1988. These consist of a list of exclusion criteria together with some positive cystoscopic features (Table 9.2). There is no universally agreed histological standard for diagnosing IC on bladder biopsy. However, biopsies are useful to exclude other pathology, including malignancy. Typical features of IC seen on cystoscopic examination include:

- subepithelial petechial haemorrhages (glomerulations)
- splotchy haemorrhages
- linear cracking of the mucosa
- white urothelial scars
- ulceration.

Treatment

Many different treatments have been tried for IC, with little sustained success. Proposed systemic treatments include antihistamines, heparin, amitriptyline and pentosan polysulphate. Pentosan polysulphate is a synthetic glycosaminoglycan analogue and augments the protective mucous layer of the bladder. Many patients with IC have been

Table 9.2
Criteria for diagnosing interstitial cystitis

Automatic inclusions	Automatic exclusions
• Hunner's ulcer	• <18 years of age
	• Bladder tumour
	• Radiation cystitis
	• Tuberculous cystitis
	• Bacterial cystitis
	• Cyclophosphamide cystitis
	• Vaginitis
	• Urethral diverticulum
	• Lower genital tract malignancy
	• Active genital herpes
	• Diurnal frequency <5 times
	• Nocturia <2 times
	• Bladder calculus
	• Detrusor overactivity
	• Capacity >400 ml

Positive factors
- Glomerulations at cystoscopy
- Low-compliance bladder
- Pain on bladder filling/ relieved on voiding

shown to have an improvement in symptoms following cystodistension. Unfortunately, any beneficial effects are short-lived.

The treatment with the most evidence to support its use is instillation therapy with dimethyl sulphoxide (DMSO, an industrial solvent). The treatment regimen is easy and inexpensive to perform on an outpatient basis, providing the patient can manage to self-catheterize. A significant improvement can be expected in over 50% of patients with early IC.[5]

> Instillation therapy with DMSO benefits women with interstitial cystitis as it is easy to perform on an outpatient basis and is inexpensive. Over 50% of patients notice a significant improvement

In a small Danish follow-up study over three years, monthly instillation of sodium hyaluronate solution (Cystistat, Pliva Pharma) showed benefit in approximately two-thirds of cases, and apparent recovery in 20%.[6] Furthermore, in a study of refractory cases of IC, an initial positive response in 56% at four weeks improved to 71% by week 12. Response then decreased after week 24 of treatment.[7]

King's College Hospital is currently part of an international multicentre study to assess the safety and efficacy of pelvic floor electro-stimulation in the treatment of IC. Although the results are awaited, the initial response appears very encouraging.

Finally, where other treatments fail and symptom severity is such that the patient's quality-of-life is destroyed, a urological opinion should be sought and reconstructive surgery considered. Available options include:

- partial cystectomy
- augmentation cystoplasty
- urinary diversion with or without cystectomy.

Sensory urgency

Sensory urgency is a diagnosis of exclusion made after urodynamic assessment. It consists of the symptom complex of frequency–urgency,

and occasionally urge incontinence, but with no evidence of DO on subtracted cystometry or other underlying intravesical pathology.

Diagnostic criteria

The exact diagnostic criteria are rather vague. Some authors have suggested cystometric parameters that require the volume of first sensation to occur at less than 100 ml and the bladder capacity to be less than 400 ml. These criteria are not universal and are heavily influenced by filling rate at cystoscopy. This makes it difficult to accurately estimate the prevalence of this condition but it is reported by 5–10% of women undergoing urodynamic assessment.

Tests

Diagnosis of this disorder requires a detailed history and examination, a frequency–volume chart and subtracted cystometry. Having made the diagnosis it is then important to undertake a cystoscopy and bladder biopsy to exclude other intravesical pathology.

> Diagnosis of sensory urgency is by a detailed history and examination, a frequency–volume chart and subtracted cystometry

Aetiology

The aetiology of sensory urgency is poorly understood and probably represents a group of women with more than one underlying pathology. Psychological factors may often play a role. Women with sensory urgency have been shown to have a heightened perception of bladder volume and to be more anxious than women with urodynamic stress incontinence or DO.[8] It is accepted that laboratory urodynamics can fail to detect DO during the comparatively brief period in which the patient is studied. Some patients who are labelled as having sensory urgency may therefore have unrecognized underlying DO, and ambulatory urodynamics may be an appropriate further investigation in these women.

Some women who are thought to have sensory urgency may have underlying DO; ambulatory urodynamics should confirm the correct diagnosis

Urethral problems

Introduction

The female urethra is a complex muscular tube approximately 40 mm in length. It is composed of:

- several layers of muscle
- the richly vascular submucosa
- the mucosa.

There is considerable debate as to the relative roles of different components of the muscles both within the wall of the urethra and surrounding it. These muscles help maintain continence. A number of changes occur to the urethra with age. The strength and the amount of urethral connective tissue fall because of oestrogen deficiency. This causes the support of the urethrovesical junction to weaken. In addition, urethral vascular pulsations in the submucosal plexus gradually decrease with age.

The muscles of the urethra help maintain continence, but the muscle tissue deteriorates with increasing age due to oestrogen deficiency

Urethritis

Urethritis is inflammation of the urethra leading to symptoms of frequency, urgency, dysuria and localized urethral pain. It is caused either by an infectious pathogen or by chemical irritation. Evidence of the use of causative chemical agents, such as bubble baths, vaginal deodorants and perfumed cosmetics, should be sought as part of the medical history in women with these symptoms. Responsible infectious agents include many of the microorganisms associated with sexually transmitted infections, such as herpes simplex virus, *Neisseria*

gonorrheae and *Chlamydia*. The group of organisms that typically cause acute bacterial cystitis, such as *Escherichia coli*, may also cause urethritis.

Where urethritis is suspected, appropriate cultures should be taken from the urethra and vagina as well as a midstream urine culture. Urine microscopy typically shows evidence of pyuria and bacteria.

Acute urinary retention can occur secondary to urethritis and needs to be considered. Prompt treatment with an indwelling catheter until symptoms have resolved is important in order to prevent overdistension of the bladder. Initiation of treatment with the appropriate antibiotic usually results in rapid recovery, but scarring of the urethra can result in strictures and subsequent voiding difficulties. Referral to a genitourinary medicine clinic for contact tracing and treatment of partners is important if sexually transmitted organisms are responsible. Cessation of the use of the offending chemical agent results in fairly rapid resolution of symptoms without the need for further treatment.

Urethral diverticula

Urethral diverticula are usually found in the distal third of the urethra bulging towards the vagina. They are thought to arise from inflammation in the paraurethral glands and are found mainly in parous women. The incidence of this condition is unclear but is probably around 3%. It is an increasingly seen problem, perhaps because of the recent rise in sexually transmitted infections.

Urethral diverticula are thought to arise from inflammation of the paraurethral glands. They are found mainly in parous women

Urethral syndrome

The term 'urethral syndrome' was first used in 1932,[9] but remains a very misunderstood condition. This is largely because there is no consensus on the definition or diagnostic criteria.

It usually refers to a symptom complex, often consisting of frequency–urgency with dysuria, in the absence of infection. Less commonly, sufferers describe suprapubic or perineal discomfort, or a sense of incomplete voiding.[10]

Aetiology

The aetiology is multifactorial and may include infection, atrophy, urethral spasm, psychogenic factors, and there may certainly be some overlap with interstitial cystitis in terms of epithelial dysfunction.[11] The diagnosis is one of exclusion, when UTI, DO and local pathology have been eliminated. When culture and sensitivity are repeatedly negative despite ongoing symptoms, especially in young women, it is worth considering culture for fastidious organisms, such as:

- *Chlamydia trachomatis*
- *Ureaplasma urealyticum*
- *Mycoplasma hominis.*

Cytology of the urine should be negative and the urodynamics should be normal. Cystourethroscopy is usually normal, but is undertaken to exclude chronic cystitis, trigonitis or neoplasms. The urethra should be carefully inspected to exclude urethral diverticula or urethritis.

Some authors have described outflow obstruction in association with urethral syndrome, and an associated turbulent backflow of bacteria in the urethra. In truth, as Benness describes in his review, there is a paucity of data to support the therapeutic benefits of urethral dilatation or urethrotomy.[10]

Psychogenic factors have been cited in the aetiology of the urethral syndrome, with evidence of a conversion or psychophysiological aetiology in 56 people who were assessed with a personality inventory.[12] However, a longitudinal assessment of community-dwelling women with either acute UTI or urethral syndrome found high levels of anxiety and psychological morbidity associated with symptoms – these resolved in both groups with cessation of symptoms.[13]

> Psychogenic factors, such as anxiety and psychological morbidity, are part of the aetiology of urethral syndrome

Reduction in levels of circulating oestrogen at the menopause results in urogenital atrophy, vaginal dryness and epithelial thinning (see Chapter 11). Loss of vaginal lubrication can lead to increased urethral trauma and subsequent symptoms after intercourse.

Treatment

Increasing the fluid intake to 'flush' the urinary tract through will serve only to increase urinary frequency. A daily fluid intake of 1.5 litres should be appropriate for metabolic needs, and will maintain a sufficiently dilute urine output to avoid the irritation of concentrated urine. Showering before intercourse and voiding afterwards should help prevent bacterial colonization.

Advice should be advised to avoid bath or shower additives, perfumed soaps and douches – these all serve to irritate the urethra further and therefore worsen symptoms.

> Patients with urethral syndrome should be advised not to use bath or shower additives, perfumed soaps or douches as they can irritate the urethra and makes symptoms worse

Methenamine hippurate 1 g bd (Hiprex, 3M Healthcare) is a urinary antiseptic that alkalinizes the urine, and may confer symptomatic relief.

In the presence of sterile pyuria, a long course of antibiotic effective against fastidious organisms is appropriate, eg norfloxacin, doxycycline or erythromycin.

Local application of oestrogen cream is effective in the treatment of vaginal and urethral atrophy. This will improve vaginal lubrication and reduce intercourse-related symptoms. It is possible to use a low dose of oestrogen replacement therapy in order to alleviate urogenital symptoms while avoiding the risk of endometrial proliferation, by using 0.1% oestriol cream (Ovestin, Organon).

References

1. Kelleher CJ, Cardozo LD, Khullar V et al. Symptom scores and subjective severity of urinary incontinence. *Neurourol Urodyn* 1994; **13**: 373–4.

2. Bungay G, Vessey MP, McPherson CK. Study of symptoms in middle life with special reference to the menopause. *Br Med J* 1980; **281**: 181–3.

3. Jarvis GJ. The management of urinary incontinence due to primary vesical sensory urgency by bladder drill. *Br J Urol* 1982; **54**: 374–6.

4. Parsons CL. Interstitial cystitis. In: Kursh ED, McGuire EJ (eds). *Female Urology*. Philadelphia: Lippincott, Williams and Wilkins, 1994, pp 421–38.

5. Perez-Marrero R, Emerson LE, Feltis JT. A controlled study of dimethyl sulphoxide in interstitial cystitis. *J Urol* 1988; **140**: 36–9.

6. Nordling J, Jorgensen S, Kallestrup E. Cystistat for the treatment of interstitial cystitis: a 3-year follow-up study. *Urology* 2001; **57(6 Suppl 1)**: 123.

7. Morales A, Emerson L, Nickel JC, Lundie M. Intravesical hyaluronic acid in the treatment of interstitial cystitis. *J Urol* 1996; **156**: 45–8.

8. Macauley A, Stanton S, Holmes D. Micturition and the mind: pyschological factors in the aetiology of urinary disorders in women. *Br Med J* 1987; **294**: 540–3.

9. Gallagher D, Montgomerie J, North J. Acute infections of the urinary tract and the urethral syndrome in general practice. *Br Med J* 1965; **543**: 622–4.

10. Benness C. Urethral syndrome. In: Staskin D, Cardozo LD (eds). *Textbook of Female Urology and Urogynaecology*. Oxford: Isis Medical Media, 2001, pp 919–24.

11. Parsons CL. Prostatitis, interstitial cystitis, chronic pelvic pain, and urethral syndrome share a common pathophysiology: lower urinary dysfunctional epithelium and potassium recycling. *Urology* 2003; **62**: 976–82.

12. Carson CC, Segura JW, Osborne DM. Evaluation and treatment of the female urethral syndrome. *J Urol* 1980; **124**: 609–10.

13. Sumners D, Kelsey M, Chait I. Psychological aspects of lower urinary tract infections in women. *Br Med J* 1992; **304**: 17–19.

10. Pregnancy

Prevalence
Causes of incontinence
Intervention

Pregnancy is characterized by dramatic changes in the anatomy and physiology of women, and these changes extend to the urinary tract. There is a 50% increase in the glomerular filtration rate of the kidneys, leading to an increased rate of urine production of around 90 ml per hour. In one study, 73% of pregnant women were found to have dilatation of the renal collecting systems, predominantly on the right side.[1] It has also been reported that renal volumes increase by up to 30%, which reverses in the postnatal period.[2] At the same time, the changes in the size and shape of the uterus cause compression of the bladder and a decrease in its functional capacity. Urinary frequency therefore increases.

> During preganancy the glomerular filtration rate increases by 50%, leading to an increased rate of urine production; the expandng uterus also compresses the bladder, thereby reducing its functional capacity and increasing urinary frequency

Prevalence

Stress urinary incontinence is a common feature of pregnancy, affecting 59% at 34 weeks gestation and reducing to 31% at 8 weeks postpartum.[3] There is no correlation at 12 weeks postpartum between symptoms of urodynamic stress incontinence (USI), diagnosis of USI and vaginal delivery.[4] Urodynamic investigation revealed a prevalence of 9% at 34 weeks gestation and 5% at 12 weeks postpartum.[5]

> 59% women have stress urinary incontinence at 34 weeks gestation

Detrusor overactivity (DO) is also associated with pregnancy,[6] with 18% suffering urge incontinence.[7] Around 15% have urge incontinence at three months postpartum[8] but only 7% have proven detrusor overactivity.[5]

Causes of incontinence

Pudendal neuropathy is common following childbirth, and is thought to be caused by a stretching injury. It is also seen in women with urinary incontinence (UI),[9,10] and so a causal relationship between childbirth and UI has long been assumed.[11] However, pregnancy (rather than childbirth) may be responsible. Incontinent nulliparous women have been shown to have a quantitative and qualitative reduction in the collagen content of their tissues[12] where no evidence of neuromuscular damage exists. In the Nuns Study, 50% of (predominantly postmenopausal) nuns complained of UI; 30% of these complained of stress incontinence, 24% had urge incontinence and 35% had mixed symptoms. Therefore, in the absence of obstetric trauma, UI is more commonly seen to be of a stress rather than an urge type.[13]

It is possible that neuromuscular damage and connective tissue deficiency are co-contributors in the aetiology of UI. Among primigravid women, those with excessive bladder-neck mobility have the highest risk of postpartum urinary incontinence.[14] It seems likely that connective tissue damage is a 'prerequisite', and that neuromuscular damage contributes to the aetiology of USI.

> Primigravid women with excessive bladder-neck mobility appear to have the highest risk of post-partum incontinence

Cyclical variations in the levels of oestrogen and progesterone during the menstrual cycle have also been shown to lead to changes in urodynamic variables and lower urinary tract symptoms. Thirty-seven percent of women notice a deterioration in symptoms prior to menstruation.[15] Furthermore, progestogens have been associated with an increase in irritative bladder symptoms[16,17] and urinary incontinence in those women taking combined hormone replacement therapy.[18] The incidence of DO in the luteal phase of the menstrual cycle may be associated with raised plasma progesterone following ovulation – progesterone has been shown to antagonize the inhibitory effect of oestradiol on rat detrusor contractions.[19] This may help to explain the increased prevalence of DO found in pregnancy.

> Progestogens have been linked with an increase in urinary incontinence and irritative bladder symptoms in women taking combined HRT

Intervention

Intervention may be preventive. Elective caesarean section may prevent neuromuscular damage[9] but may not prevent postnatal UI.[4] Rather, antenatal pelvic-floor-muscle training is effective in reducing the incidence of post-partum UI.[8] Postpartum pelvic-floor-muscle training is effective in reducing the incidence of UI at one year.[20]

The highest risk factors for UI at three months postpartum are:[8]

- vaginal delivery
- multiparity
- obesity.

> Major risk factors for urinary incontinence at 3 months' postpartum are vaginal delivery, multiparity and obesity

Follow-up of a cohort of women who delivered in 1994 showed that 31.8% of those dry pre-pregnancy are now incontinent.[21] Women with increased bladder-neck mobility have an increased incidence of stress incontinence at 14 weeks postpartum, even if there is no pre-existing symptomatology.[14] However, onset of UI prior to the initial pregnancy is the best predictor of incontinence 5–7 years later.[21] Caesarean section remains protective, but less so than at three months postpartum, with a relatively greater effect with increasing parity. The effect is particularly pronounced if the caesarean section is undertaken prelabour.[22] The most important risk factors for neuromuscular damage in labour appear to be:

- increased fetal size
- prolonged second stage
- episiotomy
- forceps delivery.[23]

'Routine' episiotomy was introduced in the UK in the 18th Century and has been advocated to prevent severe perineal tears and preserve sexual function. Review of five randomized controlled trials of the use of routine and selective episiotomy reveals that sexual function is poorer in the routine group, with no difference in the prevalence of UI and no difference in pelvic-floor-muscle strength.[24] Ventouse delivery is less traumatic than forceps, but its use has not been shown to be associated with a reduced incidence of UI or neuromuscular damage.[25]

> Important risk factors for neuromuscular damage during labour are:
> - increased fetal size
> - prolonged second stage
> - episiotomy
> - forceps delivery

References

1. Hoffmann L, Behm A, Auge A. Changes in the kidney and upper urinary tract in the normal course of pregnancy. Results of a sonographic study. *Z Urol Nephrol* 1989; **82**: 411–17.
2. Christensen T, Klebe JG, Bertelsen V, Hansen HE. Changes in renal volume during normal pregnancy. *Acta Obstet Gynecol Scand* 1989; **68**: 541–3.

3. Mason L, Glenn S, Walton I, Appleton C. The prevalence of stress incontinence during pregnancy and following delivery. *Midwifery* 1999; **15**:120–8.

4. Chaliha C, Khullar V, Stanton SL et al. Urinary symptoms in pregnancy: Are they useful for diagnosis? *Br J Obstet Gynaecol* 2002; **109**: 1181–3.

5. Chaliha C, Bland JM, Monga A et al. Pregnancy and delivery: a urodynamic viewpoint. *Br J Obstet Gynaecol* 2000; **107**: 1354–9.

6. Cutner A. The urinary tract in pregnancy. MD Thesis: University of London, 1993.

7. Cutner A, Cardozo LD, Benness CJ. Assessment of urinary symptoms in early pregnancy. *Br J Obstet Gynaecol* 1991; **98**: 1283–6.

8. Wilson PD, Herbison RM, Herbison GP. Obstetric practice and the prevalence of urinary incontinence three months after delivery. *Br J Obstet Gynaecol* 1996; **103**: 154–61.

9. Snooks SJ, Setchell M, Swash M, Henry MM. Injury to innervation of pelvic floor sphincter musculature in childbirth. *Lancet* 1984; **324**: 546–50.

10. Smith AR, Hosker GL, Warrell DW. The role of pudendal nerve damage in the aetiology of genuine stress incontinence in women. *Br J Obstet Gynaecol* 1989; **96**: 29–32.

11. Sultan AH, Kamm MA, Hudson CN. Pudendal nerve damage during labour: prospective study before and after childbirth. *Br J Obstet Gynaecol* 1994; **101**: 22–8.

12. Keane DP, Sims TJ, Abrams P et al. Analysis of collagen status in premenopausal nulliparous women with genuine stress incontinence. *Br J Obstet Gynaecol* 1997; **104**: 994–8.

13. Buchsbaum GM, Chin M, Glantz C et al. Prevalence of urinary incontinence and associated risk factors in a cohort of nuns. *Obstet Gynecol* 2002; **100**: 226–9.

14. King JK, Freeman RM. Is antenatal bladder neck mobility a risk factor for postpartum stress incontinence? *Br J Obstet Gynaecol* 1998; **105**: 1300–7.

15. Hextall A, Bidmead J, Cardozo L, Hooper R. Hormonal influences on the human female lower urinary tract: a prospective evaluation of the effects of the menstrual cycle on symptomatology and the results of urodynamic investigation. *Neurourol Urodyn* 1999; **18**: 282–3.

16. Burton G, Cardozo LD, Abdalla H et al. The hormonal effects on the lower urinary tract in 282 women with premature ovarian failure. *Neurourol Urodyn* 1992; **10**: 318–19.

17. Cutner A, Burton G, Cardozo LD et al. Does progesterone cause an irritable bladder? *Int Urogynaecol J* 1993; **4**: 259–61.

18. Benness C, Gangar K, Cardozo LD, Cutner A. Do progestogens exacerbate urinary incontinence in women on HRT? *Neurourol Urodyn* 1991; **10**: 316–18.

19. Elliot RA, Castleden CM. Effect of progestagens and oestrogens on the contractile response of rat detrusor muscle to electrical field stimulation. *Clin Sci* 1994; **87**: 342.

20. Morkved S, Bo K. Effect of postpartum pelvic floor muscle training in prevention and treatment of urinary incontinence: a one-year follow up. *Br J Obstet Gynaecol* 2000; **107**: 1022–8.

21. Wilson PD, Herbison P, Glazener C et al. Obstetric practice and urinary incontinence 5–7 years after delivery. *Neurourol Urodyn* 2002; **21**: 284–300.

22. Groutz A, Rimon E, Peled S. Caesarean section: Does it really prevent the development of postpartum stress urinary incontinence? A prospective study of 363 women one year after their first delivery. *Neurourol Urodyn* 2004; **23(1)**: 2–6.

23. Handa VL, Harris TA, Ostergard DR. Protecting the pelvic floor: obstetric management to prevent incontinence and pelvic organ prolapse. *Obstet Gynecol* 1996; **88**: 470–8.

24. Lede RL, Belizan JM, Carroli G. Is routine use of episiotomy justified? *Am J Obstet Gynecol* 1996; **174**: 1399–402.

25. Sultan AH, Kamm MA, Hudson CN, Bartram CI. Third degree obstetric anal sphincter tears: risk factors and outcome of primary repair. *Br Med J* 1994; **308**: 887–91.

11. Ageing, urogenital symptoms and hormone replacement therapy

Background
Epidemiology
Oestrogen receptors and hormonal factors
Urogenital atrophy
Lower urinary tract function
Lower urinary tract symptoms
Oestrogens in the management of incontinence
Conclusion

Background

Symptoms of urogenital atrophy are a manifestation of oestrogen withdrawal following the menopause, and may appear many years after the last menstrual period.[1] Oestrogen deficiency following the menopause is known to cause atrophic changes within the urogenital tract[2] and is associated with urinary symptoms, such as:

- frequency
- urgency
- nocturia
- incontinence
- recurrent infection.

Symptoms of urogenital atrophy occur because of oestrogen withdrawal following the menopause; they may appear many years after the last menstrual period

These may coexist with symptoms of vaginal atrophy, such as dyspareunia, itching, burning and dryness.

The role of oestrogen replacement in the treatment of these symptoms of urogenital atrophy has still not been clearly defined despite several randomized trials and widespread clinical use. This chapter presents an overview of the pathogenesis and management of urogenital symptoms and the role of oestrogen replacement therapy.

Symptoms of urogential atrophy often coexist with the symptoms of vaginal atrophy

Epidemiology

Increasing life expectancy has led to an increasingly elderly population and it is now common for women to spend one-third of their lives in the oestrogen-deficient postmenopausal state.[3] The average age of women going through the menopause is 50 years, although there is some cultural and geographical variation.[4] Postmenopausal women comprise 15% of the population in industrialized countries. In this cohort there is a predicted growth rate of 1.5% over the next 20 years.

The prevalence of symptomatic urogenital atrophy is difficult to estimate since many women accept the changes as being an inevitable consequence of the ageing process and do not seek help. It has been estimated that 10–40% of all postmenopausal women are symptomatic,[5] although only 25% are thought to seek medical help. In addition, vaginal symptoms associated with urogenital atrophy are reported by two out of three women by the age of 75 years.[6]

10–40% of postmenopausal women are symptomatic, but because they see the symptoms as an unavoidable part of ageing, only 25% actually seek medical help

Oestrogen receptors and hormonal factors

Oestrogen is known to have an important role in the function of the lower urinary tract throughout adult life, and oestrogen and progesterone receptors have been demonstrated in the:

- vagina
- urethra
- bladder
- pelvic floor musculature.[7–10]

> There are oestrogen and preogesterone receptors in the vagina, urethra, bladder and pelvic floor muscles

Oestrogen receptors are expressed in the epithelium of the urethra, vagina and trigone of the bladder.[11] They are not expressed in the dome of the bladder, thus reflecting its different embryological origin. The pubococcygeous and the musculature of the pelvic floor have also been shown to be oestrogen-sensitive.[12,13]

Androgen and progesterone receptors

In addition to oestrogen receptors, both androgen and progesterone receptors are expressed in the lower urinary tract, although their role is less clear. Progesterone receptors are expressed inconsistently, having been reported in the bladder, trigone and vagina. Their presence may be dependent on oestrogen status. In addition, whilst androgen receptors are present in both the bladder and urethra, their role has not yet been defined.[14]

Urogenital atrophy

Withdrawal of endogenous oestrogen at the menopause results in well-documented climacteric symptoms, such as hot flushes and night sweats, in addition to the less commonly reported symptoms of urogenital atrophy. Symptoms do not usually develop until several years after the menopause when levels of endogenous oestrogens fall below the level

required to promote endometrial growth.[15] This temporal relationship would suggest oestrogen withdrawal as the cause.

Vaginal symptoms

> Vaginal dryness is often the first reported symptom of urogenital atrophy. Pruritis, dyspareunia and discharge are also noted

Vaginal dryness is commonly the first reported symptom of urogenital atrophy and is caused by a reduction in mucus production within the vaginal glands. Atrophy within the vaginal epithelium leads to thinning and an increased susceptibility to infection and mechanical trauma. Following the menopause, glycogen depletion within the vaginal mucosa leads to a decrease in lactic acid formation by Döderlein's lactobacillus and a consequent rise in vaginal pH. The pH increases from around 4, to between 6 and 7. This allows bacterial overgrowth and colonization with Gram-negative bacilli, thus compounding the effects of vaginal atrophy and leading to symptoms of vaginitis, such as:

- pruritis
- dyspareunia
- discharge.

Oestrogens

> The symptoms of urogenital atrophy do not present until the levels of endogenous oestrogen are lower than that required to promote endometrial proliferation

Symptoms of urogenital atrophy do not occur until the levels of endogenous oestrogen are lower than that required to promote endometrial proliferation.[16] Consequently, it is possible to use a low dose of oestrogen replacement therapy in order to alleviate urogenital symptoms while also avoiding the risk of endometrial proliferation and removing the need to provide endometrial protection with progestogens.[17] The dose of oestradiol commonly used in systemic oestrogen replacement is usually 25–100 μg. However, studies investigating the use of oestrogens in the management of urogenital symptoms have shown that 8–10 μg of vaginal oestradiol is effective.[18] Thus, only 10–30% of the dose used to treat vasomotor symptoms may be effective in the management of urogenital symptoms. Since 10–25% of women receiving systemic hormone replacement therapy still experience the symptoms of urogenital atrophy,[19] low-dose local preparations may have an additional beneficial effect.

A recent review of oestrogen therapy in the management of urogenital atrophy has been performed by the Hormones and Urogenital Therapy (HUT) Committee.[20] Meta-analysis of 10 placebo-controlled trials confirmed the significant effect of oestrogens in the management of urogenital atrophy. Oestrogen is efficacious in the treatment of urogenital atrophy and low-dose vaginal preparations are as effective as systemic therapy.

> Low-dose vaginal preparations of oestrogen are just as efficacious as systemic therapy at treating urogenital atrophy

Lower urinary tract function

Oestrogens play an important role in the continence mechanism, with bladder and urethral function becoming less efficient with age.[21] Elderly women have been found to have:

- a reduced flow rate
- increased urinary residuals
- higher filling pressures
- reduced bladder capacity
- lower maximum voiding pressures.[22]

Oestrogens may affect continence by increasing urethral resistance, raising the sensory threshold of the bladder or by increasing α-adrenoreceptor sensitivity in the urethral smooth muscle, thereby increasing tone.[23, 24]

> Elderly women tend to have a reduced flow rate, increased urinary resistance, higher filling pressures, reduced bladder capacity and lower maximum voiding pressures

In addition, exogenous oestrogens have been shown to increase the number of intermediate and superficial cells in the vagina of postmenopausal women.[25] These changes have also been demonstrated in the bladder and urethra.[26]

Bladder function

Oestrogen receptors, although absent in the transitional epithelium of the bladder, are present in the areas of the trigone that have undergone squamous metaplasia.[24] Oestrogen is known to have a direct effect on detrusor function – oestradiol has been shown to reduce the amplitude and frequency of spontaneous rhythmic detrusor contractions.[27] There is also evidence that it may increase the sensory threshold of the bladder in some women.[28]

> Oestradiol reduces the amplitude and frequency of spontaneous rhythmic detrusor contractions. It may also increase the sensory threshold in some women

Urethra

Oestrogen receptors have been demonstrated in the squamous epithelium of both the proximal and distal urethra.[24] Oestrogen has been shown to improve the maturation index of urethral squamous epithelium.[29] It has been suggested that oestrogen increases urethral closure pressure and improves pressure transmission to the proximal urethra, both of which promote continence.[30–33]

Lower urinary tract symptoms

Epidemiological studies have implicated oestrogen deficiency in the aetiology of lower urinary tract symptoms. Seventy percent of women relate the onset of urinary incontinence to their final menstrual period.[2] Lower urinary tract symptoms have been shown to be common in postmenopausal women attending a menopause clinic, with 20% complaining of severe urgency and almost 50% complaining of stress incontinence.[34]

> Of the postmenopausal women attending a menopause clinic, approximately 20% complained of severe urgency and nearly 50% complained of stress incontinence

Urge incontinence in particular is more prevalent following the menopause and the prevalence would appear to rise with increasing years of oestrogen deficiency.[35]

There is, however, conflicting evidence regarding the role of oestrogen withdrawal at the time of the menopause. Some studies have shown a peak incidence in perimenopausal women[36,37] whilst other evidence suggests that many women develop incontinence at least 10 years prior to the cessation of menstruation, with significantly more premenopausal women than postmenopausal women being affected.[15, 38]

Urinary tract infection

Urinary tract infection is also a common cause of urinary symptoms in women of all ages. This is a particular problem in the elderly with a reported incidence of 20% in the community and over 50% in institutionalized patients.[39, 40] Pathophysiological changes, such as impairment of bladder emptying, poor perineal hygiene and both faecal and urinary incontinence, may partly account for the high prevalence observed. In addition, as previously described, changes in the vaginal flora due to oestrogen depletion lead to colonization with Gram-negative bacilli, which, as well as causing local irritative symptoms, also act as uropathogens. These microbiological changes may be reversed with oestrogen replacement following the menopause, offering a rationale for treatment and prophylaxis.

> Urinary tract infection is common in the elderly – this is likely to be due to impairment of bladder emptying, poor perineal hygiene, and faecal and urinary incontinence

Oestrogens in the management of incontinence

Oestrogen preparations have been used for many years in the treatment of urinary incontinence,[41,42] although their precise role remains controversial. Many of the studies performed have been uncontrolled observational series examining the use of a wide range of different preparations, doses and routes of administration. The inconsistent use of progestogens to provide endometrial protection is a further confounding factor making interpretation of the results difficult.

In order to clarify the situation, a meta-analysis from the HUT Committee has been reported.[43] Of 166 articles identified that were published in English between 1969–92, only six were controlled trials and 17 were uncontrolled series. Meta-analysis found an overall significant effect of oestrogen therapy on subjective improvement in all women and for women with urodynamic stress incontinence (USI) alone. However, when assessing objective fluid loss there was no significant effect. Maximum urethral closure pressure was found to increase significantly with oestrogen therapy, although this outcome was influenced by a single study showing a large effect.[44]

A further meta-analysis performed in Italy has analysed the results of randomized controlled clinical trials on the efficacy of oestrogen treatment in postmenopausal women with urinary incontinence.[45] A search of the literature (1965–96) revealed 72 articles, of which only four were considered to meet the meta-analysis criteria. There was a statistically significant difference in subjective outcome between oestrogen and placebo, although there was no difference in objective or urodynamic outcome. The authors conclude that this difference could be relevant, although the studies may have lacked objective sensitivity to detect this.

Stress incontinence

In addition to the studies included in the HUT meta-analysis, several authors have also investigated the role of oestrogen therapy in the management of USI only. Oral oestrogens have been reported to increase the maximum urethral pressures and to lead to symptomatic improvement in 65–70% of women,[46,47] although other work has not confirmed this.[16,48]

A recently reported meta-analysis has helped determine the role of oestrogen replacement in women with USI.[49] Of the papers reviewed, 14 were non-randomized studies, six were randomized trials (of which four were placebo-controlled), and two were meta-analyses. Interestingly, symptomatic or clinical improvement was only noted in the non-randomized studies. There was no such effect noted in the randomized trials. The authors conclude that currently the evidence would not support the use of oestrogen replacement alone in the management of USI.

From the available evidence, oestrogen does not appear to be an effective treatment for USI, although it may have a synergistic role in combination therapy.

> Oestrogen therapy alone does not seem to be an effective treatment for USI; however, it may have a synergistic role in combination therapy

Urge incontinence

Oestrogens have been used in the treatment of urinary urgency and urge incontinence for many years, although there have been few controlled trials to confirm their efficacy. To try to clarify the role of oestrogen therapy in the management of women with urge incontinence, a meta-analysis of the use of oestrogen in women with symptoms of 'overactive bladder' has been reported by the HUT Committee.[50] In a review of 10 randomized placebo-controlled

trials, oestrogen was found to be superior to placebo (when considering symptoms of urge incontinence, frequency, and nocturia). Vaginal oestrogen administration was found to be superior for symptoms of urgency.

> Oestrogen is suitable for treating women with urge incontinence, with vaginal administration being superior for symptoms of urgency

In those taking oestrogens there was also a significant increase in first sensation and bladder capacity when compared with placebo.

Selective oestrogen receptor modulators

A recent development in hormonal therapy has been the development of selective oestrogen receptor modulators (SERMs), see Table 11.1. These drugs have oestrogen-like actions in maintaining bone density and in lowering serum cholesterol, but have anti-oestrogenic effects on the breast[51] and do not cause endometrial stimulation.[52] In theory, partial oestrogen antagonists may lead to a down-regulation of oestrogen receptors in the urogenital tract and consequently cause an increase in lower urinary tract symptoms and symptomatic urogenital atrophy.

Table 11.1
Some licensed SERMs

- Clomiphene
- Tamoxifen
- Toremifene
- Raloxifene

Early work would suggest that some SERMs in development, eg levormeloxifene and idoxifene, might increase the risk of urogenital prolapse,[53] although there were some methodological problems noted in the study. However, in another analysis of three randomized, double-blind, placebo-controlled trials investigating raloxifene in 6926 postmenopausal women, drugs appeared to have a protective effect – fewer treated women had surgery for urogenital prolapse: 1.5% vs 0.75% ($p<0.005$).[54]

At present, the long-term effect of SERMs on the urogenital tract remains to be determined and there are few data regarding effects on urinary incontinence and urogenital atrophy

Conclusions

Oestrogens are known to have an important physiological effect on the female lower genital tract throughout adult life, leading to symptomatic, histological and functional changes. Urogenital atrophy is the manifestation of oestrogen withdrawal following the menopause, presenting with vaginal and/or urinary symptoms. The use of oestrogen replacement therapy has been examined in the management of lower urinary tract symptoms as well as in the treatment of urogenital atrophy. Only recently has this treatment been subjected to randomized placebo-controlled trials and meta-analysis.

Oestrogen therapy alone has been shown to have little effect in the management of USI. When considering the irritative symptoms of urinary urgency, frequency and urge incontinence, oestrogen therapy may be of benefit, although this may simply represent reversal of urogenital atrophy rather than a direct effect on the lower urinary tract.

Finally, low-dose vaginal oestrogens have been shown to have a role in the treatment of urogenital atrophy in postmenopausal women and would appear to be as effective as systemic preparations.

References

1. Iosif CS. Effects of protracted administration of oestriol on the lower genitourinary tract in postmenopausal women. *Acta Obstet Gynaecol Scand* 1992; **251**: 115–20.

2. Iosif C, Bekassy Z. Prevalence of genitourinary symptoms in the late menopause. *Acta Obstet Gynaecol Scand* 1984; **63**: 257–60.

3. *American National Institute of Health Population Figures*. Washington, DC: US Treasury Department/NIH, 1991.

4. Research on the menopause in the 1990's. Report for a WHO Scientific Group. *WHO Technical Report Series 866*. Geneva: WHO, 1994.

5. Greendale GA, Judd JL. The menopause: Health implications and clinical management. *J Am Geriatr Soc* 1993; **41**: 426–36.

6. Samsioe G, Jansson I, Mellstrom D, Svanborg A. The occurrence, nature and treatment of urinary incontinence in a 70 year old population. *Maturitas* 1985; **7**: 335–43.

7. Cardozo LD. Role of oestrogens in the treatment of female urinary incontinence. *J Am Geriatr Soc* 1990; **38**: 326–8.

8. Iosif S, Batra S, Ek A, Astedt B. Oestrogens receptors in the human female lower urinary tract. *Am J Obstet Gynaecol* 1981; **141**: 817–20.

9. Batra SC, Fossil CS. Female urethra, a target for oestrogen action. *J Urol* 1983; **129**: 418–20.

10. Batra SC, Iosif LS. Progesterone receptors in the female urinary tract. *J Urol* 1987; **138**: 130–4.

11. Blakeman PJ, Hilton P, Bulmer JN. Mapping oestrogen and progesterone receptors throughout the female lower urinary tract. *Neurourol Urodyn* 1996; **15**: 324–5.

12. Ingelman-Sundberg A, Rosen J, Gustafsson SA. Cytosol oestrogen receptors in urogenital tissues in stress incontinent women. *Acta Obstet Gynaecol Scand* 1981; **60**: 585–6.

13. Smith P. Oestrogens and the urogenital tract. *Acta Obstet Gynecol Scand* 1993; **72**: 1–26.

14. Blakeman PJ, Hilton P, Bulmer JN. Androgen receptors in the female lower urinary tract. *Int Urogynaecol J* 1997; **8**: S54.

15. Samicoe G. Urogenital ageing – a hidden problem. *Am J Obstet Gynecol* 1998; **178**: S245–S249.

16. Wilson PD, Faragher B, Butler B et al. Treatment with oral piperazine oestrone sulphate for genuine stress incontinence in postmenopausal women. *Br J Obstet Gynaecol* 1987; **94**: 568–74.

17. Mettler L, Olsen PG. Long term treatment of atrophic vaginitis with low dose oestradiol vaginal tablets. *Maturitas* 1991; **14**: 23–31.

18. Smith P, Heimer G, Lindskog, Ulmsten U. Oestradiol releasing vaginal ring for treatment of postmenopausal urogenital atrophy. *Maturitas* 1993; **16**: 145–54.

19. Smith RJN, Studd JWW. Recent advances in hormone replacement therapy. *Br J Hosp Med* 1993; **49**: 799–809.

20. Cardozo LD, Bachmann G, McClish D et al. Meta-analysis of oestrogen therapy in the management of urogenital atrophy in postmenopausal women: second report of the Hormones and Urogenital Therapy Committee. *Obstet Gynaecol* 1998; **92**: 722–7.

21. Rud T, Anderson KE, Asmussen M et al. Factors maintaining the urethral pressure in women. *Invest Urol* 1980; **17**: 343–7.

22. Malone-Lee J. Urodynamic measurement and urinary incontinence in the elderly. In: Brocklehurst JC (ed). *Managing and Measuring Incontinence. Proceedings of the Geriatric Workshop on Incontinence, July 1988*. Geriatric Medicine.

23. Versi E, Cardozo LD. Oestrogens and lower urinary tract function. In Studd JWW, Whitehead MI (eds). *The Menopause*. Oxford: Blackwell Scientific, 1988, pp 76–84.

24. Kinn AC, Lindskog M. Oestrogens and phenylpropanolamine in combination for stress incontinence. *Urology* 1988; **32**: 273–80.

25. Smith PJB. The effect of oestrogens on bladder function in the female. In Campbell S (ed). *The Management of the Menopause and Postmenopausal Years*. Carnforth: MTP, 1976, pp 291–8.

26. Samsioe G, Jansson I, Mellstrom, D, Svandborg A. Occurance, nature and treatment of urinary incontinence in a 70 year old female population. *Maturitas* 1985; **7**: 335–42.

27. Shenfield OZ, Blackmore PF, Morgan CW *et al*. Rapid effects of oestriol and progesterone on tone and spontaneous rhythmic contractions of the rabbit bladder. *Neurourol Urodyn* 1998; **17**: 408–9.

28. Fantl JA, Wyman JF, Anderson RL *et al*. Post menopausal urinary incontinence: comparison between non-oestrogen and oestrogen supplemented women. *Obstet Gynaecol* 1988; **71**: 823–8.

29. Bergman A, Karram MM, Bhatia NN. Changes in urethral cytology following oestrogen administration. *Gynaecol Obstet Invest* 1990; **29**: 211–13.

30. Rud T. The effects of oestrogens and gestogens on the urethral pressure profile in urinary continent and stress incontinent women. *Acta Obstet Gynaecol Scand* 1980; **59**: 265–70.

31. Hilton P, Stanton SL. The use of intravaginal oestrogen cream in genuine stress incontinence. *Br J Obstet Gynaecol* 1983; **90**: 940–4.

32. Bhatia NN, Bergman A, Karram MM *et al*. Effects of oestrogen on urethral function in women with urinary incontinence. *Am J Obstet Gynecol* 1989; **160**: 176–80.

33. Karram MM, Yeko TR, Sauer MV *et al*. Urodynamic changes following hormone replacement therapy in women with premature ovarian failure. *Obstet Gynaecol* 1989; **74**: 208–11.

34. Cardozo LD, Tapp A, Versi E et al. The lower urinary tract in peri- and postmenopausal women. In: *The Urogenital Defiency Syndrome*. Bagsverd, Denmark: Novo Industri AS, 1987, pp 10–17.

35. Kondo A, Kato K, Saito M *et al*. Prevalence of hand washing incontinence in females in comparison with stress and urge incontinence. *Neurourol Urodyn* 1990; **9**: 330–1.

36. Thomas TM, Plymat KR, Blannin J *et al*. Prevalence of urinary incontinence. *Br Med J* 1980; **281**: 1243–5.

37. Jolleys JV. Reported prevalence of urinary incontinence in a general practice. *Br Med J* 1988; **296**: 1300–2.

38. Burgio KL, Matthews KA, Engel B. Prevalence, incidence and correlates of urinary incontinence in healthy, middle aged women. *J Urol* 1991; **146**: 1255–9.

39. Sandford JP. Urinary tract symptoms and infection. *Anna Rev Med* 1975; **26**: 485–505.

40. Boscia JA, Kaye D. Assymptomatic bacteria in the elderly. *Infect Dis Clin North Am* 1987; **1**: 893–903.

41. Salmon UL, Walter RI, Gast SH. The use of oestrogen in the treatment of dysuria and incontinence in postmenopausal women. *Am J Obstet Gynecol* 1941; **14**: 23–31.

42. Youngblood VH, Tomlin EM, Davis JB. Senile urethritis in women. *J Urol* 1957; **78**: 150–2.

43. Fantl JA, Cardozo LD, McClish DK and the Hormones and Urogenital Therapy Committee. Oestrogen therapy in the management of incontinence in postmenopausal women: A meta-analysis. First report of the Hormones and Urogenital Therapy Committee. *Obstet Gynaecol* 1994; **83**: 12–18.

44. Henalla SM, Hutchins CJ, Robinson P, Macivar J. Non-operative methods in the treatment of female genuine stress incontinence of urine. *Br J Obstet Gynaecol* 1989; **9**: 222–5.

45. Zullo MA, Oliva C, Falconi G *et al*. Efficacy of oestrogen therapy in urinary incontinence. A meta-analytic study. *Minerva Ginecol* 1998; **50**: 199–205.

46. Caine M, Raz S. The role of female hormones in stress incontinence. In: *Proceedings of the 16th Congress of the International Society of Urology*. Amsterdam 1973.

47. Rud T. The effects of oestrogens and gestagens on the urethral pressure profile in urinary continent and stress incontinent women. *Acta Obstet Gynaecol Scand* 1980; **59**: 265–70.

48. Walter S, Wolf H, Barlebo H, Jansen H. Urinary incontinence in postmenopausal women treated with oestrogens: a double-blind clinical trial. *Urol Int* 1978; **33**: 135–43.

49. Ahmed Al-Badr, Ross S, Soroka D, Drutz HP. What is the available evidence for hormone replacement therapy in women with stress urinary incontinence? *J Obstet Gynaecol Can* 2003; **25**: 567–74.

50. HUT Committee Report, 2001. Unpublished.

51. Park WC, Jordan VC. Selective oestrogen receptor modulators (SERMs) and their roles in cancer prevention. *Trends Mol Med* 2002; **8**: 82–8.

52. Silfen SL, Ciaccia AV, Bryant HU. Selective oestrogen receptor modulators: tissue selectivity and differential uterine effects. *Climacteric* 1999; **2**: 268–83.

53. Hendrix SL, McNeeley SG. Effect of selective oestrogen receptor modulators on reproductive tissues other than endometrium. *Ann NY Acad Sci* 2001; **949**: 243–50.

54. Goldstein SR, Neven P, Zhou L *et al*. Raloxifene effect on frequency of surgery for pelvic floor relaxation. *Obstet Gynaecol* 2001; **98**: 91–6.

12. Pads, catheters and containment

Pads
Aids
Odour control
Devices
Catheters
Summary

Incontinence can be cured or significantly improved in most women providing they are appropriately investigated and treated. However, some women may not wish to undergo medical or surgical intervention. There are also a number of women for whom a cure may be impossible. For this group, containment with pads, devices or even catheters may be the most appropriate therapy.

> Women who cannot be cured of their incontinence are still suitable for containment therapy with pads or catheters

Reported figures[1] estimate the overall cost of incontinence to the NHS at £354 million, with the cost continuing to rise.[2] Continence products are one of the biggest expenditures for the NHS today.

Products available are numerous, but it is important to match the product to the individual's personal needs, wishes and social circumstances. It is difficult even for a specialist continence nurse to keep up with the choice available. Companies are constantly changing and developing their products, endeavouring to ensure that their products suit the requirements of the users.

Pads

The pad is the most common and the most readily available form of containment. The market of reusable and disposable products has grown tremendously. In 1974 Bill Kylie, an Australian, launched an oblong absorbent pad that became the forerunner of the disposable pad industry. There are few quality trials to assess pads, and many products have frequently been replaced before the results are published.

> Pads should only be used as a temporary measure while investigations are being undertaken or treatment is awaited. They should be used where containment is a priority

Pads should not be used as an alternative to effective continence promotion strategies. They should really be a temporary measure while investigations are undertaken or treatment is awaited. Pads should only be used as treatment in the severely incontinent person where containment will be a priority.

The ideal pad should be reliable, simple to use and aesthetically pleasing to the user. Every pad has been produced to deal with different types of incontinence:

- Small pads are for light incontinence or frequent changes.
- Large pads are for the containment of heavy incontinence or where toileting is not an option.[3]

Pads can either be disposable or reusable. There is no strong evidence that one is more effective than the other. The advantages and limitations of reusable and disposable products are outlined in Table 12.1. The commonest problem with disposable pads is that they can become bulky and the covering can even become separated if they are not replaced when needed.[4]

Disposable pads

Many forms of disposable pads exist:

- The body-worn pad attaches the pad to the pant and enables use with normal underwear.

Table 12.1
Advantages and disadvantages of different types of incontinence pads

	Advantages	Limitations
Reusables	● Cannot be torn apart	● Require washing
	● Retain better shape	● Initial capital outlay
	● Do not break up	● May be unacceptable to users (especially if
	● More design options	menstruating or faecally incontinent)
	● Independence from supply system	
	● Eliminate storage	
	● Can be reused if dry	
Disposables	● Flexibility to match users requirements	● Tendency for pulp compression
	● No laundry	● Tendency for pulp break-up
	● Materials better suited to faecal incontinence	● Can be torn apart

● The pad and pant system is recommended for women who are able to undertake toileting.

● All-in-one pads can be particularly effective in containing urine and poorly formed faeces. They are mainly used for the severely disabled, bed-fast patient or when toileting is difficult.

● The pouch pad is held in place in the pouch of a washable pair of pants with a waterproof gusset.

● The bed pad is designed as bed protection when there is the added risk of soiling or when a body-worn pad is not suitable.

> The five main types of disposable pad are the body-worn pad, the pad and pant system, all-in-one pads, the pouch pad, and the bed pad

Reusable pads

The decision whether or not to use reusable incontinence products rather than disposables is a complex one that will depend on individual needs and preferences. The availability of suitable laundry facilities is an important factor.[4]

Aids

Over a thousand items, ranging from special toilet seats to assist toilet training to odour-control products are listed in The United Kingdom Continence Foundation Product Directory.[5]

Aiding toileting

Simple measures may make a huge difference, especially for women with urgency and urge incontinence. These include:

● fewer layers of loose-fitting clothes

● light slippery fabrics (which cling less and may be easier to adjust)

● short vests, shirts or blouses (which are less likely to get in the way)

● easy-to-launder fabrics that do not retain odour

● thumb or hand loops attached to waistbands (which can help women with limited manual dexterity)

● suitable clothes (which can disguise pad and catheter use).

> Many simple measures – eg easy-to-launder clothing fabrics that do not retain odour, suitable clothes to disguise pad or catheter use, and loose-fitting clothes – can help women with urgency and urge incontinence

Commodes

Commodes come with a variety of functions, including adjustable-height legs and removable arms and backs.[6] Many are designed to look like well-designed chairs and appear as part of the ordinary furniture. Chemical toilets/commodes need emptying less often.

Odour control

People who have incontinence frequently become obsessed that they smell. All that is needed is:

- reassurance
- good personal hygiene
- prompt disposal of products
- prevention of urinary infection.

Devices

In recent years there has been a wide variety of new continence devices developed.[7] Although interest continues with clinicians and patients, many of the devices have never made it onto the market or have been removed from the market shortly after release. Some products are available on the Internet, but until these products become more widely available, they will continue to be limited to specialist units in controlled trials.

The main aims of specifically designed continence devices have been to manage stress incontinence – with or without prolapse. These include:

- external urinary collection devices or appliances
- intravaginal devices that support the bladder neck
- occlusion devices that are:
  - external to the meatus
  - intraurethral.

There are limited devices for faecal incontinence.

Catheters

Catheters are used for bladder drainage when there are defects or obstruction in the lower urinary tract

Catheters are widely used for effective bladder drainage, either temporarily or permanently, when physiological and anatomical defects or obstruction of the lower urinary tract are present. When dealing with incontinence, all other possibilities for treatment or management must be explored following appropriate investigation.

Catheter insertion falls into two main groups:

- urethral
  - indwelling
  - intermittent, eg clean intermittent self-catheterization (CISC)
- suprapubic.

> The two insertion categories of catheter are urethral (either indwelling or intermittent) and suprapubic

Urethral catheterization

The urethral catheter is the most frequently used catheter as it can be quickly and easily inserted. Urethral catheterization is an accepted aseptic procedure and should be undertaken under the guidance of strict local hospital or community infection-control policies.

Catheter selection

Designs and materials

All catheters in the UK must now conform to British Standards following reports that some catheters were associated with cytotoxicity.[8] Plastic or PVC and latex rubber are for short-term use only. They tend to attract surface deposits, causing encrustation and fractures within the catheter. Plastic catheters are also rigid and uncomfortable, causing bladder spasm and bypassing.[9] Improvements on the latex catheter include 'siliconizing' the surface of the catheter producing a lubricant effect to facilitate insertion. Latex has also been coated in Teflon (polytetrafluoroethylene, PTFE) to make it more inert and to give it a smoother surface to reduce urethritis and encrustation.

For long-term use, silicone elastomer-encapsulated (coated) latex catheters are recommended. Silicone reduces the incidence of trauma, urethritis and encrustation. Hydrogel catheters (eg Biocath, Bard) are similar to silicone catheters but they become smoother when hydrated.

> Short-term catheters should be made from Teflon-coated latex to reduce urethritis and encrustation; long-term catheters tend to be made from silicone elastomer-encapsulated latex, which reduces the incidence of trauma, urethritis and encrustation

A comparison of urethral reactions to 100% silicone catheters, hydrogel-coated catheters and siliconized latex catheters demonstrated that:

- 100% silicone catheters had the lowest incidence of urethral inflammation
- hydrogel catheters proved to be the most superior in preventing encrustation
- the siliconized latex catheters were the least effective in both urethral inflammation and the prevention of encrustation.[10]

Catheter size and length

Catheters are measured in 'French' gauge (Fg) or 'Charriere' (Ch) units. This is the measurement of the external circumference in millimetres, which is approximately equal to three times the external diameter, depending on the catheter material. Catheters used in women should range from size 12Ch to 16Ch, with a small balloon.

Catheters are available in three lengths:
- male 41–44 cm
- female 22–26 cm
- paediatric ~30 cm.

For women who are obese, the shorter female catheters may cause discomfort.

> For obese women, a male-length catheter may be more suitable

Catheter-associated problems

Infection

Urinary tract infection is the most frequent complication with long-term indwelling catheters. Most catheter users will have bacteria in the urine within three days.[11] Infections can be difficult to eradicate due to the growth of bacterial populations as an adherent biofilm on the catheter surface. Common pathogens, such as *Escherichia coli*, are eliminated from the urine but persist in the biofilm and restart the cycle of infection.[12]

Leakage, bypassing and blockage

The incidence of catheter blockage and bypassing in long-term catheterization is around 48% for blockage and around 37% for bypassing.[13] Large catheter, detrusor spasm, blockage, debris or bladder calculus are all reasons for catheter failure. The use of a smaller catheter will help reduce the incidence of abnormal bladder contractions.

> There is blockage in around 48% of long-term catheters and bypassing in approximately 37%

To protect against blockage, an adequate fluid intake, greater than 1.5 litres, is recommended. Factors that may trigger catheter blockage include:[14]

- acidic fluids (eg fruit juice)
- calcium-rich foods and supplements
- alcohol, which may lead to dehydration.

> Acidic fluids (such as fruit juice), calcium-rich foods and alochol can all trigger catheter blockage

Although debris in the urine is almost certain in any woman who has a long-term catheter, general mobilization can protect against it accumulating and subsequently blocking the drainage eyes of the catheter. In women who are immobile, regular assisted change of position is advocated. Constipation should be avoided as this can cause leakage and bypassing. Straining on defecation may cause expulsion of the catheter.

Suprapubic catheterization

For women who have intractable incontinence, suprapubic catheterization is the preferred route. This is the insertion of a catheter into the bladder wall just above the symphysis pubis. It can be inserted under a general or local anaesthetic.

For long-term use a Foley catheter made of an inert material, eg hydrogel, should be used. Medium-sized catheters, size 14Ch–16Ch are ideal. They can be changed every three months with little effort once a 'track' or 'fistula' has been formed. This change may be needed more frequently if they are prone to encrustation and blockage. Suprapubic catheters, as with urethral catheters, drain urine via a 'closed system' into a drainage bag. However, valves are used as an alternative for some women.

> For women who have intractable incontinence, suprapubic catheterization is preferred to urethral catheterization

Catheter drainage bags

Drainage bags connected directly to a catheter should have a non-return valve to prevent any refluxing of urine once it has entered the bag, and should be changed once a week to reduce the risk of infection caused by biofilm build-up.[15] Women should be offered a small body-worn drainage bag – the so-called 'leg bag'. Manufacturers have developed a wide variety of methods to keep the drainage bags in place, including:

- fabric ties
- Velcro straps
- 'sporran' belts
- integrated pockets or sleeves.

Leg bags, however, do not have the capacity for drainage of urine whilst the user is asleep. So that the closed system is not broken, a 'night bag' is fitted to the tap of the 'leg bag' so the urine can flow from the smaller leg bag into the larger two-litre night bag.

Valves

The use of valves, instead of continuous drainage bags, is increasing in popularity. The release of the valve will be dependent on the fluid intake and bladder capacity. By releasing the valve around every three to four hours it can maintain bladder tone, as the bladder will fill and empty as under normal conditions. It is certainly more discreet for the user. However, it is contraindicated if any of the following are present:

- reduced manual dexterity
- dementia
- uncontrolled detrusor overactivity
- poor renal function.

Clean intermittent self-catheterization

Clean intermittent self-catheterization (CISC) is a technique taught to patients (although carers can also be taught if necessary) to facilitate bladder emptying. This may relieve overflow incontinence. It is also useful in treating women with idiopathic or neurogenic detrusor overactivity, enabling them to instil anticholinergic drugs intravesically.[16] Proper assessment, reassurance and continuing support are vital if women are to be motivated to perform catheterization themselves.

> Clean intermittent self-catheterization is a technique taught to patients or carers to facilitate bladder emptying and relieve overflow incontinence

Catheter types

PVC is frequently used for CISC, with a lubricant to facilitate insertion. Plastic catheters can be reused, for up to one week, as long as the user is infection-free and has a good technique. Self-lubricating (hydrophilic) catheters have been developed with evidence that the higher the osmolality within the catheter, the less friction there is on insertion.[17] Unfortunately they are expensive and single-use only.

Ultimately, catheter choice will depend on the individual and what is available. Most women will use a size 10Ch–12Ch. It is not unreasonable for women to use a longer 'male' length if they find it easier. If women have difficulty in directing the catheter into their urethra, there are aids to help guide them.

Summary

No one product suits everyone and unfortunately some products are not available to everyone. Holistic patient assessment is the key to achieving containment of incontinence by product use. Regular review will ensure whether the patient's needs are being met or not. For those who have to rely on pads and pants, devices, aids or catheters, the right product or mode of containment must be suitable for the individual.

References

1. Department of Health. *Modernising Health and Social Services: National Priorities Guidance. 1999/00–2001/02.* London: Department of Health, 1998.

2. Prescription Cost Analysis – England – 1999 (Department of Health, 2000). *Continence Foundation Newsletter* 2001; Issue 6.

3. Shepherd A, Blannin J. The role of the nurse. In: Mandelstam D (ed). *Incontinence and its Management, 2nd edition.* Beckenham: Croom Helm, 1986.

4. Norris C, Cottenden A, Ledger D. Underpad overview. *Nurs Times* 1993; **89**: 21.

5. *Continence Products Directory 2nd edition.* London: The Continence Foundation, 1996.

6. Association of Continence Advisers. *Directory of Aids to Toileting, 1st edition.* London, 1985.

7. Anders K. Non medical management of incontinence. In: Cardozo L, MacLean AB (eds). *Incontinence in Women.* London: RCOG Press 2002, pp 225–48.

8. Ruuta M, Alfhan O, Anderson LC. Cytotoxicity of latex urinary catheters. *Br J Urol* 1985; **57**: 82–7.

9. Blannin J., Hobden J. The Catheters of Choice. *Nurs Times* 1980; **76**: 2092–3.

10. Talji M, Korpela A, Jarvi K. Comparison of urethral reactions to full silicone, hydrogel coated and siliconised latex catheters. *BJ Urol* 1990; **6**: 652–7.

11. Bach D, Hess EA, Prauge CH. Prophylaxis against encrustation and urinary tract infection with indwelling transurethral catheters. *Urol Nephrol* 1990; **2**: 25–32.

12. Stickler DI, Chawia IC. The role of antiseptics in the management of patients with long term indwelling bladder catheters. *J Hosp Infect* 1987; **10**: 219–28.

13. Kohler-Ockmore J, Feneley RC. Long-term catheterization of the bladder: prevalence and morbidity. *Br J Urol* 1996; **33**: 347–51.

14. Burr RG, Nuseibeh IM. Urinary catheter blockage depends on urine pH, calcium and rate of flow. *Spinal Cord* 1997; **35**: 521–5.

15. Rogers J, Norkett DI, Bracegirdle P *et al.* Examination of biofilm formation and risk of infection associated with the use of urinary catheters with leg bags. *J Hosp Infect* 1996; **32**: 105–15.

16. O'Flynn KJ, Thomas DG. Intravesical instillation of oxybutinin hydrochloride for detrusor hyperreflexia. *Br J Urol* 1993; **72**: 566–70.

17. Walker L, Telanderm M, Sullivan L. The importance of osmolality in hydrophilic urethral catheters: a crossover study. *Spinal Cord* 1997; **35**: 229–33.

13. Frequently asked questions

Is urinary incontinence normal?

Involuntary loss of urine is never 'normal'. It may well be transient and self-limiting (such as with a urinary tract infection in the elderly), or short-lived (such as during the latter stages of pregnancy). Persistent symptoms indicate pathology and warrant investigation and treatment.

Doesn't incontinence only affect old people?

Although the prevalence of detrusor overactivity increases linearly with age,[1] the peak age for urodynamic stress incontinence is around age 50.[2] Urinary incontinence can affect the broadest age range. The effects on the quality-of-life of the woman are age-dependent. However, age is not a reason to dictate any particular management strategy, which should be individualized according to the background, wishes and beliefs of the woman.

My mother had incontinence. Does that mean I will become incontinent?

Data indicate the presence of hereditary factors in the development of urinary incontinence in women[3] – there is an increased risk for any incontinence (stress and mixed type) and severe symptoms. Where a mother has incontinence, there is an increased risk in her daughter [Any: odds ratio (OR) 1.4, 95% confidence interval (CI)1.3–1.6; Severe: OR 2.2, CI 1.4–3.3]. If the grandmother as well as the mother has/had incontinence, the risk is increased further (OR 2.9, CI 1.1–7.6).

Whether or not the basis of these associations is strictly genetic is not known. It is more likely that inheritance of this condition is multifactorial, with bad habits passed on from mother to daughter across generations.

If I drink lots of mineral water, will that protect my bladder?

There is no evidence to support the suggestion that excessive levels of fluid intake will improve bladder function. Rather, a high fluid intake merely exacerbates urgency–frequency and urge incontinence.

The use of a frequency–volume chart (bladder diary) is a cheap, straightforward and effective way of ensuring optimal fluid intake of around 1.5 litres per day. Frequency–volume charts are both valid and useful, with good correlation between patients' recordings on the chart and collected urine volume.[4]

In the Norwegian EPINCONT study[5] of 27 936 women, potentially modifiable lifestyle factors were assessed for their association with urinary incontinence. Former and current smoking, obesity and tea intake were all significantly associated with incontinence. Although alcohol and coffee intake were not shown to be associated with incontinence, caffeine and alcohol are known to be diuretics and bladder irritants, and can be expected to exacerbate urinary urgency and frequency.

I do a lot of sports – surely that will help?

There is a high prevalence of stress and urge incontinence in elite athletes,[6] which is significantly associated with the presence of an eating disorder. Elite athletes tend to have very low body fat and are often amenorrhoeic over a long period. Urogenital atrophy may therefore become a problem. Unless training is specifically targeted at the pelvic floor muscles, sports programmes are unlikely to help beyond reducing obesity and encouraging cessation of smoking.

Some sports may be considered to have a detrimental effect on the pelvic floor. Road running, trampolining and aerobics are high-impact activities – a retrospective study confirms that athletes who compete in high-impact sports are more likely to report urinary incontinence whilst undertaking their activity than athletes participating in low-impact sports.[7] This effect did not, however, seem to predispose to higher rates later in life.

Can anything be done to help?

The majority of cases of urinary incontinence can be cured or significantly improved if properly investigated, diagnosed and treated. Quality-of-life assessments have shown improvements after appropriate treatment.[8]

I have tried pelvic floor exercises. What else is available?

Although properly supervised pelvic-floor-muscle training has been shown to be effective in the treatment of urodynamic stress incontinence and mixed incontinence,[9] it is not an effective treatment for detrusor overactivity. Detrusor overactivity is better treated with bladder drill[10] and anticholinergic medication.[11] It is common practice for pelvic-floor exercises to be described by midwives after delivery, and it is certainly the case that fewer women have incontinence postnatally if they undertake pelvic-floor exercises properly.[12] However, in our experience, these exercises are often incorrectly performed unless taught and reviewed by a specialist physiotherapist, continence advisor or specialist nurse. It is worth bearing in mind that over a 5–7-year period, there will be a significant incidence of onset or resolution of symptoms in affected women.

Women who have undertaken pelvic-floor-muscle training, and in whom no satisfactory amelioration of symptoms has been achieved, can be reassured that effective surgical techniques are available.[13, 14]

Will I have to take tablets forever?

The treatment of detrusor overactivity (DO) is, as previously stated, behavioural and pharmacological. These modalities provide symptomatic relief but do not alter the pathological process, which is idiopathic in most women. The treatment is therefore expected to be of long duration.

The natural history of DO is of worsening and remitting symptoms. Although the newer delivery systems (extended-release, patch or intravesical instillations) have a lower incidence of side-effects, these can still be troubling in some women. Therefore, the use and dose of medication should be reviewed and altered as the need changes.

How can I stop getting so many attacks of cystitis?

Women should be advised to maintain an adequate fluid intake of 1.5 litres per day, or a slightly increased amount after exertion or on hot days. Cranberry, as either juice or tablets, will act as an effective, safe and pleasant prophylaxis. Showering before, and voiding after, intercourse should be advised – where symptoms are strongly intercourse-related, consider taking a single dose of an antibiotic, such as norfloxacin, and changing contraception from a diaphragm and spermicidal jelly (if appropriate). Postmenopausal women should be offered oestrogen cream to use intravaginally on a regular basis; and where necessary, all women should be counselled as to the option of using prophylactic antibiotics if all investigations are normal.

References

1. Milsom I, Abrams P, Cardozo L et al. How widespread are the symptoms of overactive bladder and how are they managed? A population-based prevalence study. *BJU Int* 2001; **87**: 760–6.

2. Hannestad YS, Rortveit G, Sandvik H, Hunskaar S. A community-based epidemiological survey of female urinary incontinence: the Norwegian EPINCONT study. Epidemiology of incontinence in the County of Nord-Trondelag. *J Clin Epidemiol* 2000; **53**: 1150–7.

3. Hannestad Y, Lie RT, Rortveit G, Hunskaar S. Female urinary incontinence – running in the family? *Neurourol Urodyn* 2003; **22**: 448.

4. Palnæs Hansen C, Klarskov P. The accuracy of the frequency-volume chart: comparison of self-reported and measured volumes. *Br J Urol* 1998; **81**: 709–11.

5. Hannestad YS, Rortveit G, Daltveit AK, Hunskaar S. Are smoking and other lifestyle factors associated with female urinary incontinence? The Norwegian EPINCONT Study. *Br J Obstet Gynaecol* 2003; **110**: 247–54.

6. Bø K, Borgen JS. Prevalence of stress and urge urinary incontinence in elite athletes and controls. *Med Sci Sports Exerc* 2001; **33**: 1797–802.

7. Nygaard IE. Does prolonged high-impact activity contribute to later urinary incontinence? A retrospective cohort study of female Olympians. *Obstet Gynecol* 1997; **90**: 718–22.

8. Bidmead J, Cardozo L, McLellan A *et al*. A comparison of the objective and subjective outcomes of colposuspension for stress incontinence in women. *Br J Obstet Gynaecol* 2001; **108**: 408–13.

9. Hay-Smith EJ, Bo Berghmans LC, Hendriks HJ *et al*. Pelvic floor muscle training for urinary incontinence in women. *Cochrane Database Syst Rev* 2001; **1**: CD001407.

10. Jarvis GJ, Millar DR. Controlled trial of bladder drill for detrusor instability. *Br Med J* 1980; **281**: 1322–3.

11. Anderrson K-E *et al*. Pharmacological treatment of urinary incontinence. In Abrams P, Cardozo LD, Khoury S, Wein A (eds). *Incontinence. 2nd International Consultation on Incontinence July 1–3, 2001*. Health Publication, 2002, pp 479–511.

12. Glazener CM, Herbison GP, Wilson PD *et al*. Conservative management of persistent postnatal urinary and faecal incontinence: randomised controlled trial. *Br Med J* 2001; **323**: 593–6.

13. Alcalay M, Monga A, Stanton SL. Burch colposuspension: a 10–20 year follow up. *Br J Obstet Gynaecol* 1995; **102**: 740–5.

14. Ward KL, Hilton P; UK and Ireland TVT Trial Group. A prospective multicenter randomized trial of tension-free vaginal tape and colposuspension for primary urodynamic stress incontinence: two-year follow-up. *Am J Obstet Gynecol* 2004; **190**: 324–31.

Appendix A: The King's Health Questionnaire

1. How would you describe your health at the present?

Please tick one answer

Very good ○

Good ○

Fair ○

Poor ○

Very poor ○

2. How much do you think your bladder problem affects your life?

Please tick one answer

Not at all ○

A little ○

Moderately ○

A lot ○

Below are some daily activities that can be affected by bladder problems.

How much does your bladder problem affect you?

We would like you to answer every question, simply tick the box that applies to you

	1 Not at all	2 Slightly	3 Moderately	4 A lot
3. Role limitations				
A. Does your bladder problem affect your household tasks (cleaning, shopping, etc)?	○	○	○	○
B. Does your bladder problem affect your job, or your normal daily activities outside the home?	○	○	○	○

	1 Not at all	2 Slightly	3 Moderately	4 A lot
4. Physical/social limitation				
A. Does your bladder problem affect your physical activities (eg going for a walk, running, sport, gym, etc)?	○	○	○	○

B. Does your bladder problem affect your ability to travel? ○ ○ ○ ○

C. Does your bladder problem limit your social life? ○ ○ ○ ○

D. Does your bladder problem limit your ability to see and visit friends? ○ ○ ○ ○

	0 Not Applicable	1 Not at all	2 Slightly	3 Moderately	4 A lot
5. Personal relationships					
A. Does your bladder problem affect your relationship with your partner?	○	○	○	○	○
B. Does your bladder problem affect your sex life?	○	○	○	○	○
C. Does your bladder problem affect your family life?	○	○	○	○	○

	1 Not at all	2 Slightly	3 Moderately	4 Very much
6. Emotions				
A. Does your bladder problem make you feel depressed?	○	○	○	○
B. Does your bladder problem make you feel anxious or nervous?	○	○	○	○
C. Does your bladder problem make you feel bad about yourself?	○	○	○	○

	1 Never	2 Sometimes	3 Often	4 All the time
7. Sleep/energy				
A. Does your bladder problem affect your sleep?	○	○	○	○
B. Does your bladder problem make you feel worn out and tired ?	○	○	○	○

8. Do you do any of the following?   **If so how much?**

	1 Never	2 Sometimes	3 Often	4 All the time
A. Wear pads to keep dry?	○	○	○	○
B. Be careful how much fluid you drink ?	○	○	○	○
C. Change your underclothes because they get wet?	○	○	○	○
D. Worry in case you smell?	○	○	○	○

We would like to know what your bladder problems are and how much they affect you? From the list below choose only those problems that you have at present. Leave out those that don't apply to you.

How much do the following affect you?

Frequency: going to the toilet very often

        1. A little   2. Moderately   3. A lot

         ○   ○   ○

Nocturia: getting up at night to pass urine

        1. A little   2. Moderately   3. A lot

         ○   ○   ○

Urgency: a strong and difficult-to-control desire to pass urine

        1. A little   2. Moderately   3. A lot

         ○   ○   ○

Urge incontinence: urinary leakage associated with a strong desire to pass urine

        1. A little   2. Moderately   3. A lot

         ○   ○   ○

Stress incontinence: urinary leakage with physical activity, eg coughing, running

        1. A little   2. Moderately   3. A lot

         ○   ○   ○

Nocturnal enuresis: wetting the bed at night

        1. A little   2. Moderately   3. A lot

         ○   ○   ○

Intercourse incontinence: urinary leakage with sexual intercourse

        1. A little   2. Moderately   3. A lot

         ○   ○   ○

Waterworks infections

        1. A little   2. Moderately   3. A lot

         ○   ○   ○

Bladder pain

        1. A little   2. Moderately   3. A lot

         ○   ○   ○

To calculate scores:

PART 1

1) General Health Perceptions

Very good   1

Good   2

Fair   3

Poor   4

Very poor   5

Score = [(Score to Q1 − 1)/4] × 100

2) Incontinence Impact

Not at all   1

A little   2

Moderately   3

A lot   4

Score = [(Score to Q2 − 1)/3] × 100

PART 2

Individual scores as recorded at the top of each column of possible responses

3) Role limitations

    Score = {[(Scores to Q 3A + 3B) − 2]/6} × 100

4) Physical limitations

    Score = {[(Scores to Q 4A + 4B) − 2]/6} × 100

5) Social limitations

    [If 5C ≥ 1] Score = {[(Score to Q 4C + 4D + 5C) − 3]/9} × 100

    [If 5C = 0] Score = {[(Score to Q 4C + 4D) − 2]/6} × 100

6) Personal relationships

    [If 5A+5B ≥2] Score = {[(Scores to Q 5A + 5B) − 2]/6} × 100

    [If 5A+5B =1] Score = {[(Scores to Q 5A + 5B) − 1]/3} × 100

    [If 5A+5B =0] Treat as missing value

7) Emotions

> Score = {[(Score to Q 6A + 6B + 6C) − 3]/9} X 100

8) Sleep/energy

> Score = {[(Scores to Q 7A + 7B) − 2]/6} x 100

9) Severity measures

> Score = {[(Scores to Q 8A + 8B + 8C + 8D) − 4]/12} x 100

PART 3

Scale	Score
Omitted	0
A little	1
Moderately	2
A lot	3

Appendix B: Levels of evidence[1, 2]

I   Systematic review of all relevant RCTs

IIA   One randomized controlled trial (RCT) – low probability of bias and high probability of causal relationship

IIB   One randomized controlled trial (RCT)

IIIA   Well designed controlled trials (no randomization)

IIIB   Cohort or case–control studies

IIIC   Multiple time series or dramatic results in uncontrolled experiments

IV   Expert opinion (traditional use)

Grades of recommendations

A   A systematic review of RCTs or a body of evidence consisting principally of studies rated as 1 directly applicable to the target population and demonstrating overall consistency of results

B   A body of evidence including studies rated as 2A directly applicable to the target population and demonstrating overall consistency of results *or*

     Extrapolated evidence from studies rated as 1

C   A body of evidence including studies rated as 2B directly applicable to the target population and demonstrating overall consistency of results *or*

     Extrapolated evidence from studies rated as 2

D   Evidence level 3 or 4 *or*

     Extrapolated evidence from studies rated as 2

1. Hadorn DC, Baker D, Hodges JS, Hicks N. Rating the quality of evidence for clinical practice guidelines. *J Clin Epidemiol* 1996; **49**: 749–54.

2. Harbour R, Miller J. A new system for grading recommendations in evidence based guidelines. *Br Med J* 2001; **323**: 334–6.

Appendix C: Useful contacts

The International Continence Society

ICS Office, Southmead Hospital, Bristol BS10 5NB

Tel: 0117 950 3510
Fax: 0117 950 3469
Email: info@icsoffice.org
Web: www.icsoffice.org

The International Continence Society is centrally involved in standardization, education and development of all areas of continence promotion and pelvic floor dysfunction. The website provides links to useful documents, to abstracts presented at the annual meetings, and to many organizations around the world who are involved in patient care or research. The Society is truly multidisciplinary, comprising doctors, nurses, physiotherapists, continence advisors, scientists and other professionals who are involved in the care of women with lower urinary tract dysfunction and pelvic floor dysfunction.

The Continence Foundation

307 Hatton Square, 16 Baldwin Gardens, London EC1N 7RJ

Tel: 0845 345 0165
Web: www.continence-foundation.org.uk

The website is a good resource for practitioners with an interest in the management of incontinence. It is fully vetted by a Development Committee – comprising a consultant urologist, a consultant gynaecologist, a consultant colorectal surgeon, a physiotherapist, a continence services manager and a geriatrician.

A helpline (open 9.30–1.00, Monday to Friday), staffed by continence nurse specialists, takes enquiries from healthcare professionals as well as the public.

International Urogynaecology Association

www.iuga.org

The International Urogynecological Association is an international organization committed to promoting and exchanging knowledge regarding the care of women with urinary and pelvic floor dysfunction. Membership of IUGA consists of obstetricians/gynaecologists, urologists, urogynaecologists, biomedical engineers, physiotherapists, nurses and other professionals who are involved in the care of women with lower urinary tract dysfunction.

*In*contact

United House, North Road, London N7 9DP

Tel: 0870 770 3246
Fax: 0870 770 3249
Email: info@incontact.org
Web: www.incontact.org/

*In*contact is the UK organization for people with bladder and bowel problems. Formed in 1989 by a group of patients and health professionals, the organization provides information and support to people affected by these common conditions, as well as their carers and the health professionals who look after them.

Association of Chartered Physiotherapists in Women's Health (ACPWH)

c/o The Chartered Society of Physiotherapy 4 Bedford Row, London WC1R 4ED

Tel: 020 7306 6666
Web: www.womensphysio.com

ACPWH represent chartered physiotherapists who specialize in Women's Health in the UK and abroad. There are over 600 members, whose work includes the treatment of conditions such as urinary and faecal incontinence and back and pelvic problems in women who are pregnant or have recently had a baby.

Healthcare professionals and members of the public who wish to be put in contact with a local ACPWH member should write to the Membership Secretary at the above address. Contact the Book and Leaflet Secretary, also at the above address, for a list of leaflets on relevant subjects.

National Electronic Library for Health Specialist Library – Women's Health

Web: www.whsl.org.uk/urogyn

The Women's Health Specialist Library aims to provide all professionals involved in the care of women with access to the best current knowledge to support clinical decisions; to regularly search, evaluate and categorize

resources currently available online; to signpost users to high-quality, evidence-based resources; to provide a monthly electronic newsletter highlighting new additions to the library; to provide the women's health knowledge base for the NHS Electronic Health Record; and to work with NHS Direct to ensure the public receives appropriate health information.

The Cochrane Incontinence Review Group

Web: www.otago.ac.nz/cure

The Cochrane Incontinence Review Group is a Collaborative Review Group of the Cochrane Collaboration, an international organization dedicated to disseminating information on the best available evidence in healthcare. The website provides access to the Cochrane reviews related to incontinence.

Index

(Abbreviations used USI = urodynamic stress incontinence; UTI = urinary tract infection)
Page numbers in *italics* refer to information that is shown only in a table or diagram.